Living With Sickle Cell

The Inside Story

2nd Edition

JUDY GRAY JOHNSON

Editor: Ava Teherani
Front and Back Cover Design: Juan Roberts, Creative Lunacy
Interior Design: John Sibley, Rock Solid Productions

ISBN: 978-0-9967162-08
Library of Congress Control Number: 2015949689

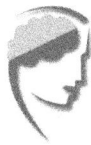

KNOWLEDGE POWER BOOKS
www.knowledgepowerbooks.com

Printed in the United States of America

Dedication

In recent years, there have been improvements and new discoveries in diagnosis, treatment, and research. I have lived for more than seventy-two years with sickle cell disease and even today, I wonder how I have endured so much pain throughout my life. For these reasons, I dedicate this book to:

- Florence Neal Cooper Smith, a pioneer of sickle cell awareness in Richmond, Virginia
- Other sickle cell sufferers and their families

These people are pioneers for the advocacy of improved care for sickle cell patients. Their united mission is to bring awareness of sickle cell disease to the lay community and to educate health care providers.

Acknowledgements

To my daughter, Dr. Loree Anitra Johnson, I thank you for being my eyes and ears to the world. As you read these pages, you will learn even more than you know about the strong lineage into which you were born. I would also like to thank my aunts, Amanda Gray Perry and Louise Gray Guinyard, both of whom graduated from South Carolina State College. They had an entrepreneurial side as well. Aunt Amanda is an artist who sold many of her paintings. Aunt Louise became an antique dealer.

I also want to acknowledge my sister, Dr. Rosemary Gray, who went on to become Vice President of Special Services and Equity at McNeese State University, where she also serves as the Americans with Disability Coordinator and the Title I Coordinator.

I would also like to pay tribute to the following family members, who are now deceased:

- My mother, Janie Turner Gray, who attained an eighth grade education and never earned more than minimum wage.
- My father, Therman Gray Sr., who completed fifth grade, yet became known for his mechanical ability.
- My brother, Therman Gray Jr., who completed his B S degree from Claflin University.
- My brother, Donald Wayne Turner, who passed away at an early age with heart problems, but not before serving his country in the United States Army.
- My sister, Linda Gray Lyons, who completed high school at sixteen. Although we were born only eighteen months apart, she served as a surrogate mother to me during what was a physically and emotionally painful childhood.
- My grandfather, Harry Gray, who could not read or

write, yet became known throughout the state of South Carolina as one of the best mechanics around. Until his death in 1961, while working with his son Therman Sr., he used that knowledge to not only support his family, but to send three daughters and two grandchildren to college.

- My grandmother, Lula Rountree Gray, who completed sixth grade. Although a top student, opportunities did not exist for her to continue her education. She was the "glue" that held the family together. When Granddaddy was faced with the challenge of assembling a complex piece of farm equipment used to cut and bind hay for transport, my grandmother read him the directions.

- My aunt, Ruth Gray Matthews, also a South Carolina State College graduate, who passed away at thirty-two due to complications arising from multiple sclerosis.

- My uncles, Paul Turner, Eldridge Turner, and Hoyate Turner Sr. They all finished their high school education and served with distinction in the United States military. During my early years, my uncles served as the support system that provided our family with shoes on our feet, food on the table, and gifts at Christmas.

Linking the members of my family is a thread of perseverance. We neither complained nor did we quit. We overcame life's obstacles by "repositioning" ourselves whenever necessary.

I want to give a special thank you to Leroy Williams, Jr. my co-author on the 1st Edition of *Living with Sickle Cell Disease: The Struggle to Survive.*

Table of Contents

Introduction

Sickle cell disease is the most misunderstood disease ever. While more and more people have heard of the term or perhaps know of someone that "has it," the depth of knowledge and understanding does not exist. After reading my book you will come away with not only being able to define the disease, but to begin to see the disease for what it really is. My story is really the story of millions of sicklers worldwide. The only difference is name, date, and locations of events. My family is their family. My encounters and interactions with friends, doctors, and hospitals are their experiences as well. There are exceptions to everything. You will find perhaps 5% of sicklers with different and better support systems. The 95% of us that remain are desperately seeking your willingness to know and understand this disease - not just topically, but internally as well.

You will discover that sickle cell disease is NOT "what you see is what you get!" Keep in mind that we truly are survivors. Every day that we awake, we are mentally mapping out a plan to get through the day. This supersedes everything else in our lives. So, while we may look normal, please know that there is a "struggle" inside that is not understood by most. It is important for you, the reader, to know this and to feel this struggle.

As you grow in understanding, what will you do with this newfound knowledge? It is my hope that you, regardless of your ethnicity, will seek out a hematologist to have a HEMOGLOBIN ELECTROPHORESIS blood test done. Afterward, sit down with your hematologist and have them explain the results to you and what it means for YOU and your family. This is something that each family member should do. We can all look back within our community and know of someone who was either ill or died from some mysterious illness. There was a tendency to just call it by some general term when we did not know the true cause. IT IS IMPORTANT for everyone to know their medical history for many reasons: impact on the quality of life physically, mentally, and socially; what constitutes a disability; to seek out information about the disabled as it applies to your state and community; to take advantage of services that may be available to those who are "different"; how to engage the community in providing for all its citizens; to determine how the disabled can be an active participant in their care (short-term & long-term); and to develop a need for self sufficiency as much as humanly possible.

At present, there is no cure except it has been proven that a bone marrow/stem cell transplant can cure sickle cell disease. However, in order to proceed, the patient should ask lots of questions. This is a risky procedure in which many more trials are needed in order to work out the "kinks" in the system. The problem that the community needs to understand is that there is a low "donor" pool among various ethnic groups, especially the African American and Latino communities. What is known about this procedure is that bone marrow/stem cell transplants are very risky, and can have serious side effects, including death. For the transplant to work, the bone marrow donor should have a similar genetic type to the person receiving the bone marrow (a close match). Usually, the best donor is a brother or sister. Bone marrow/stem cell transplants are typically done only in cases of severe sickle cell disease for children who have minimal organ damage from the disease at the time of transplant.

However, going forward, this book is meant to instill an awareness of this disease and to ask you to do what you can individually to minimize the impact of this disease on society. You CAN do it.

S. C. D.

There is a monster that exists; his initials are S. C. D.
This monster is invisible
And he truly deceives.
Although he attacks,
Others find it hard to believe.
S. C. D. brings about excruciating pain.
When under attack, the victim becomes crippling and lame.
This monster is prejudiced
and leaves the voiceless with no name.
He chokes the life out of some and those struggling
to breathe he wants you also to come.
This monster is metamorphic,
He changes his shape like the gravitational curved path of an orbit.
The distorted shapes are clustered
and the unpleasantness is especially morbid.
There is a second monster that comes after the first.
In fact, this one is much worse.
As this second monster laughs and mocks
He asks, "Did you come for your NARCS?
Once we give you these then it will be time for you to leave.
We will even escort you while you're still on your knees.
Don't come back now ya hea cause if you do
we'll leave you hangin thea."
The victim cries, help me, help me, help me please...
Free me from my captor, also known as Sickle Cell Disease!

~ Tamara Holmes ~ 07/30/2015

Chapter One
My Earliest Memories of Pain

"Failure will never overtake me if my determination to succeed is strong enough.
Og Mandino

"Cut out the drama," the male nurse said to me. Had he not lobbed that verbal grenade at me while I was roaring like a bear caught in a trap, I would likely have returned fire with a fusillade of eloquent obscenities. However, I was in the most agonizing pain that I believe any human could experience. It was pure physical distress, which felt as though one hundred serrated steak knives were piercing my body from within. Those doctors and nurses could not have gotten the pain medication into my system fast enough. They were trying to administer the pain relief drugs intravenously, which had been a challenge because my veins had collapsed.

After spending an overly unnecessary amount of time trying to figure out how to connect me to that infernal IV, the medical staff decided to insert the needle into my neck. I think they called it the internal jugular vein. That's when that insensitive clod of a so-called medical professional told me to cease my audition for One Life to Live.

Well, so much for bedside manners!

It is terrible to be wheeled on a gurney into the controlled insane asylum, otherwise known as a hospital emergency room. Going in there alone, without a spouse, a child, a sibling, or a cousin, can be a frightening experience. How else will my family understand what is going on with me if they don't see or hear it firsthand from the doctors? This is true especially when a person, such as me, is a long-divorced woman within shouting distance of seventy-three years old.

As a person whom demographers charitably categorize as a senior citizen, I tend to forget a few things when my body feels like it's under attack from killer bees. For example, some of the things that I may forget to inform the doctors about, include the types of medication and dosage that have proven to be more effective for me. My brain was furiously processing a different kind of message from my screaming nerve endings. These pain indicators tended to compete for my attention that may have otherwise been directed towards the inquisitive medical personnel.

The inexplicably rude behavior exhibited by the male nurse is, unfortunately, typical of the treatment that I have encountered from a wide array of medical professionals who have treated me whenever I experience a sickle cell crisis.

If at all possible, the patient should never go to the hospital alone. Parents or caretakers should arrange for someone to take turns staying with the patient around the clock until the pain has subsided. The patient may or may not remember any details while in a crisis and the nurses may not always be as attentive as they should be. Unfortunately, too many medical personnel see tears as drug withdrawals. This is why parents, when there is not a crisis, should become familiar with all medications needed. When the patient has to go to the hospital, always have paper and pen to take notes to write down the names and positions of all persons you come in contact with. Write down all procedures done, medication dosage that was given and by whom. It's a good idea to keep this information in a notebook. Date everything!

A patient with the genetic blood disorder known as sickle cell disease lives with a condition that is characterized by red blood cells that assume an abnormal sickle shape. Normally red blood cells are shaped like small donuts. According to the United States Center for Disease Control and Prevention (CDC), healthy red blood cells are round and they move through small blood vessels to carry oxygen to all parts of the body. In sickle cell disease, the red blood cells become hard and sticky and look like a C-shaped farm tool called a sickle. The sickle cells die early, which causes a constant shortage of red blood cells. In addition, as these blood cells travel or float through small blood vessels, they can become stuck and clog blood flow throughout the human body. This can cause pain and other serious problems.

According to literature from the CDC, there are three common types of sickle cell disease. People with the HbSS form of sickle cell disease inherit two sickle cell genes, known as S, one from each parent. This is commonly called sickle cell anemia and is usually the most severe form of the disease. Another is HbSC, which is the type I have and is a milder form of sickle cell disease in which people inherit one sickle cell gene and one gene from an abnormal type of hemoglobin called C. Hemoglobin is a protein that allows red blood cells to carry oxygen to all parts of the body. Oxygen is an essential element in the survival of cells and tissue. HbS beta thalassemia is the third form. There are significant differences in disease patterns for each type of sickle cell disease. All of this may cause an increase in fetal hemoglobin, which can protect the red blood cells from becoming sickled and can cause complications.

The sickle cell disease process often results in severe anemia, oxygen deprivation, extreme pain, and poor blood circulation. Each type of sickle cell disease can cause pain episodes known as "crises" and other complications, which are disabling and debilitating.

According to the Genetic Science Learning Center at the University of Utah, the occurrences of these common types of sickle cell disease in African Americans are:

- One in 375 for HbSS;
- One in 835 for HbSC;
- One in 1,667 for HbS beta thalassemia.

In addition, one in twelve African Americans has the sickle cell trait.

Sickle cell disease was first discovered in 1910, according to the 2009 Sickle Cell Anemia Foundation Annual Report. The November 1910 issue of The Archives of Internal Medicine carried an article by James B. Herrick of Chicago. Herrick's article was called, "Peculiar Elongated and Sickle-Shaped Red Blood Corpuscles in a Case of Severe Anemia." Three months later, in the February 1911 issue of the Virginia Medical Semi-Monthly, an author erroneously identified as

R.E. Washburn, from the University of Virginia (the name should have read B.E. Washburn), published a report citing Herrick's article and used precisely the same descriptive title diagnosis with a sixteen-year-old, in order to provide some reassurance and understanding. At sixteen years old, I was a child who needed someone to tell me that everything would be okay.

As I researched material for this book, I came across the story of Henrietta Lacks, an African American woman and tobacco farmer whose cells were taken without her knowledge in 1951 as she was being treated for cervical cancer. The cancer cells became known as the HeLa line and have become one of the most important tools in medicine, vital for developing the polio vaccine, cloning, gene mapping, in vitro fertilization, and more. Henrietta's cells have been bought and sold by the billions, yet she remained unknown until the 2010 publication of her biography, *The Immortal Life of Henrietta Lacks* by Rebecca Skloot.

I found, to my shock and surprise, that Henrietta's life and mine had many parallels. Among them are that we both came from poor families, and we were both born in southwestern Virginia. (Henrietta was born in Roanoke and I was born in Gate City.) One aspect of her life particularly intrigued me: She refused to submit to a test for sickle cell disease. My question became what if she had said "yes" to the sickle cell anemia test? I wondered how science regarding sickle cell disease would have changed had Henrietta taken the test and did in fact have sickle cell disease. Was there a connection between the HeLa cell line and sickle cell anemia? Has the HeLa line in any way contributed to the understanding of sickle cell anemia? According to one scientist, experiments performed in HeLa cells have provided mechanistic insights into the way all cells work. Therefore, the results of experiments in HeLa cells have advanced our understanding of all disorders of normal cellular processes. Sickle cell anemia results from a mutation of a gene that functions only in red blood cells. Since HeLa cells were derived from cervical cells, which are very different from red blood cells, the results of experiments performed with HeLa cells are not directly related to sickle cell anemia. Hopefully, some in the medical profession will read Ms. Skloot's book and mine and become inspired to advance their research on a cure for sickle cell disease.

In my community, African-American adults discussed very little of substance with minors, probably to shelter children from life's unpleasantness. Because they had no point of reference, it was difficult for my family members to explain to me what was happening to my body physically, to assist me in understanding my disease, or even to verbalize the pain and discomfort that I was going through. I went about my life for the next forty or so years with a superficial knowledge of sickle cell disease, pushing it back in my mind until the pain flared up. I would have tried on my own to learn more, but I was afraid, especially once I learned that sickle cell disease is potentially fatal.

What could I have done differently if my aunt had sat me down and told me what that doctor told her? Truly, I will never know. What I do know is that I would never have averted the crisis—the most common complication of sickle cell disease and the top reason that people with sickle cell disease go to the emergency room or hospital. During a sickle cell crisis, blood vessels that are clogged with sickled cells cause mild to severe pain that can start suddenly and last for any length of time. During most of my life, I did not call them crises; I referred to them as pain episodes. I used to say to myself that when pain knocked on my door, there was no seat for him. However, pain told me not to worry because he had brought his own stool.

In the early years, my treatment consisted of occasional doctor's visits with instructions for my mother to apply liniment - a topical anesthetic - to the affected area. For me this meant that during many painful episodes, the pain just wore off. In later years, after my diagnosis, I was in and out of doctor's offices and hospitals as the painful crises came and went. At one point in time, the crises struck about a year apart, but as I have advanced into my sixties, they seem to have come on more rapidly every few months, with fire-like frequency. Moreover, more times than not, I have had to deal with medical personnel who seem insensitive to the pain sickle cell disease patients endure. I recall as a child suffering so badly that I would secretly wish for an amputation of whatever limb was hurting, because I thought that if the extremity were cut off, then I would experience no more pain.

Anemia is another complication that afflicts many sickle cell patients. In sickle cell disease, the red blood cells die early. Sickled cells have a lifespan of only sixteen days as compared to the normal one hundred and twenty days for healthy cells. This results in too few healthy red blood cells left to carry oxygen throughout the body. When this happens, according to the CDC, a person might undergo fatigue, irritability, dizziness and lightheadedness, a rapid heart rate, difficulty breathing, pale skin color, jaundice (yellow color to the skin and whites of the eyes), slow growth, or delayed puberty.

As a child, I often felt tired, yet I never complained of my fatigue for fear that someone might ridicule me for my sluggishness. Everyone already knew that I did not do any work around the house. So how was I going to convince anyone that I was tired? My family concluded that I was lazy, plain and simple. Somehow, no one connected my tiredness with my illness, two random factors that would not be linked until I was well into my fifties. My sluggish self-image would stay with me throughout childhood and into adulthood. Over time, I tried to understand what was happening within my body. I learned that while I did not require much sleep, I did require a lot of rest.

As a public school teacher presiding over classes of elementary and middle school students, I got very little rest during the day over the years. I spent a lot of time on my feet as I walked around the classrooms to ensure my pupils stayed on task. While the crises came and went, fatigue was a constant companion. Being tired was nothing new to me. That is who I was, because I never knew a life of not feeling tired. I knew I had to develop my own strategy for survival.

On the outside, *sicklers*—those of us with sickle cell disease—appear normal. However, behind the scenes, our constant tiredness prompts us to budget our energy as most folks budget their time or money. In addition, as a teacher, my daily routine involved waking up at four o'clock in the morning, but staying in bed to rest. After taking a shower, I would have to return to bed to rest once again. A few minutes would pass before I could gradually put on one item of clothing after another. Each day, I had to choose how I would conserve my energy in order to get through the day. Therefore, I had to be creative. I usually arrived at school at least an hour before the rest of the staff. The custodians became accustomed to my walking into the building with them. At times, I had been known to sit in the parking lot, waiting for the custodians to arrive. I did not mind this because it gave me a chance to rest.

I entered the classroom and sat at my desk, making mental observations of what I needed to do to get through the day. My checklist consisted of objectives on the chalkboard, required student materials in place, extra supplies on hand, and ensuring all equipment was operational. There was ample time for me to spread out what needed to be done and to rest in between each task before other staff members entered the building.

When most teachers left the building at the end of the school day, I remained holed up in my classroom with the door shut, resting. In my mind, I slowly replayed my day and evaluated how it had gone. I asked myself what I needed to do more of, or differently, in order to make sure I would have an easier time the next day. This also allowed me to work at my own pace grading papers and completing any other assignments the school required. On weekends, I built obligatory personal items into my schedule, along with schoolwork that I had to complete for the coming week.

I knew very well that other folks saw me as lazy, but I disregarded it without discussing my physical state of exhaustion, because I did not know that the fatigue could be related to my illness. For many years, I simply did not understand the extent to which sickle cell disease was affecting my life. With that being the case, I could not very well explain it to others.

I was married, albeit for only five years. From that union, I had a daughter, Loree. I thank God that she does not have sickle cell disease or the sickle cell trait. I raised my daughter by myself from the time when she was thirteen months old. While managing and struggling with my own health issues, I had the added physical stress of providing for her, nurturing her, and fighting to give her a first-class education. Loree went through her young life as if she were training to go to Harvard University. This would provide her with a wide range of choices in later years. Anything short of her excelling academically would have been unacceptable. I know she was fortunate to have a mother who believed that education took place well beyond the walls of the classroom.

Loree's love for travel was one that she acquired rather honestly. Her great aunt on her father's side of the family had traveled to six continents and many countries in between. My mother and I both were curious about the world, but we remained so and were unable to satisfy this curiosity, due to a life of poverty and health issues that were beyond our control. Loree earned a Ph.D. from Syracuse University and she has a thriving family practice in Los Angeles, Santa Clarita and Hermosa Beach, California.

Despite my health challenges and outward image of laziness, I taught elementary school for over forty years during my career as an educator. I retired in 2011. I earned a bachelor's and a master's degree in elementary education and special education, and I completed coursework for the doctorate in administration and supervision. I was President of the Fairfax County Federation of Teachers (FCFT) for three consecutive terms. The union represented teachers and instructional assistants who worked in the Fairfax County Public Schools, the largest school district in Virginia and the twelfth largest school district in the nation.

My life's experiences have prompted me to write this book. I have outlived the average sickle cell patient, believing that my life will serve as a purpose-driven story. Mine is a story of a search—a quest for respect, dignity, self-discovery, and finally, advocacy. This drive has enabled me to tell others how I have managed to live with the disease. However, I know that this book is not an end-all. I hope others will continue the public discussion of the disease as it affects the family, community, and the workplace.

Whenever someone asks me what has shaped my life, I respond by saying that it was shaped by living with sickle cell disease. As a child, people called me "sickly." As a young adult, people thought that I was slothful, due to my constant fatigue. Today, as a mature senior, I consider myself a survivor. I am writing this book with the hope of informing others, including medical professionals, employers, family, and friends, about my experiences, and the true nature of sickle cell disease from one woman's perspective.

It is possible to live a productive life even when your body does not want to cooperate; one just has to be creative. Because I have lived through it, I would like to share my story with sickle cell patients, their caretakers, medical professionals, and others. What follows is the story of my life. I hope this narrative will serve to assist those who, like me, suffer its intermittent pain.

Chapter Two
Liniment, "The One and Only Cure-All"

"Our greatest weakness lies in giving up. The most certain way to succeed is always to try just one more time."

Thomas A. Edison

I was born and raised in Gate City, which is the seat of Scott County, Virginia. The town is nestled in the mountains of extreme Southwestern Virginia, just north of its border with Northeastern Tennessee, and a stone's throw from Kingsport, Tennessee, which is also the closest major city. Scott County lies between the Cumberland Plateau on the northwest and the Appalachian Mountains on the southeast.

The River, a 1984 film starring Sissy Spacek and Mel Gibson, was filmed in Gate City.

Scott County is part of Appalachia, a mountainous region that stretches through thirteen states, from New York to Mississippi. When I was born in the 1940s, the entire area of Scott County suffered from economic depression. The county population was just under 27,000 people. The 1964 Appalachian Regional Commission's report to the President stated that the region was faced with a myriad of unmet needs, including food, clothing, medical care, housing, basic education, skills, jobs, hope, and dignity. Even today, Appalachia remains, to some extent, unable to shed its image as a stagnant, underdeveloped region that is lagging behind the rest of the country.

One can imagine what things were like in Scott County back in the 1940s. The line that divided black and white arbitrarily separated those who had very little from those who had considerably less. However, there was little racial tension.

Blacks and whites got along well within the community. Segregation was basically due to wealth and not race. At that time, many black families felt that a life of poverty was part of their lot in life. People wore humility on their sleeves. Very few people brought attention to themselves. They did not talk about past events, even when asked. Most households shared the perspective that what goes on inside the walls of one's home, stayed there. Under no circumstances were family members to talk about family business to outsiders. Adults rarely spoke to their children about matters that affected the community. Children, as the old saying went, were to be seen and not heard.

Among the more prominent members of Gate City's black community was Mary Wolfe Coley, who was born in 1913 and who was first educated at Prospect Elementary School, then at Slater High School in Bristol, Tennessee. She went to Morristown College in Morristown, Tennessee. Miss Mary, as many knew her, graduated as the valedictorian at all three schools. In addition to the moniker Miss Mary, Mary Wolfe Coley was also known as Mama, Mama Mary, Aunt Mary, Grandma Mary, and Mam-Maw.

Ms. Louise Dykes, also known as Aunt Weedie, was another distinguished resident. Her father was a local blacksmith, and her husband owned one of the first automobiles driven around Gate City. Aunt Weedie was known for sewing, and she produced what many folks considered the most beautiful quilts ever seen. Aunt Weedie's father was a violinist who played at various functions in the community, and the children would often dance to his music.

I can only tell you that my family associated somehow with folks like Miss Mary and Aunt Weedie, who were part of Gate City's close-knit black community.

The black community itself consisted of two hundred and fifty people. I know because I made a point of counting black households and the number of people in each one. Many black families lived in the trot, or possum trot, as it was known then. Other black families lived up on the hill, which was known as Sticktown.

Among the other landmarks in Gate City is the Church of Christ, which is more than one hundred years old. The concrete blocks used to build the church were molded from cement mixed at the building site. The pastor and the men from the community built the church. The Church of Christ's annual homecoming was held on the first Sunday of September with preaching, music, and dinner on the church grounds.

Hale's Chapel United Methodist Church was built in July 1903, on land purchased for one hundred dollars. Its members originally held worship services at Prospect Elementary School. Mary Wolfe Coley was the church pianist and superintendent of the Sunday school from 1936 to 1998. None of the pastors lived in Gate City. Their compensation for officiating services and for their travel—first via horse and buggy, then by car or train—was a weekly salary of $3.75 and a meal. Annual homecoming services at Hale's Chapel were typically held on the church grounds on the second Sunday of September.

Prospect Elementary School was the colored school in Gate City, and it also served as a community gathering place. Built in 1919, it was the only black school in Scott County. Mary Wolfe Coley was the principal at Prospect Elementary from 1936 to 1965, at which point she, like many black teachers, lost her position after the U.S. Supreme Court ordered the desegregation of public schools in 1954. From 1965 to 1980, she worked as the assistant librarian at the elementary school. She taught for forty-four years in Scott County.

A major employer in Scott County was the limestone quarry in Spiers Ferry, Virginia. Established in 1916, the quarry supplied limestone rock for the cement production plant in nearby Kingsport, Tennessee. Many Scott County residents worked in the Stanley Coal Mine. The mine was established when Clint Stanley began digging for coal with a pick, a shovel, dynamite, and blasting caps. Mr. Stanley was the father of coal mining on Cove Creek. Houses for families of coal miners were built near the mining operations.

Other industries were logging, quarries, and sand processing plants. Crafts practiced were doll and basket making. For black folks in Scott County at the time, a good job would be to work as a custodian at one of the major employers (i.e., Kingsport Press and Tennessee Eastman) in nearby Kingsport, Tennessee.

Scott County had fewer doctors at the turn of the twentieth century than it did in modern times, due to the difficulty of transportation. People had to rely on trains or horse and buggy to get around the mountainous terrain. Doctors resided in nearly every remote section of the county.

It was into this rural, impoverished milieu that I was born on January 5, 1943, to Therman and Janie Turner Gray. I was delivered into this world with the help of a midwife. Many poor people at that time used midwives to deliver their babies because the fees that a midwife charged were substantially less than those charged by doctors.

I was Therman and Janie's fourth child of five. I was named for Judy Turner Isen, who was known as Aunt Jude, the sister of my maternal great-grandfather. Aunt Jude lived in Gate City from 1870 to 1950 and was employed as a domestic for many years. Aunt Jude's home was located at the end of the aforementioned possum trot.

The hard times undoubtedly affected my family. Households across America found it difficult to recover from the Great Depression of the 1930s. By the 1940s, the United States was embroiled in World War II. Locally, things were even more difficult. Our part of Appalachia was growing substantially slower than the nation in employment and earnings. Unemployment rates for black men were twice that of whites.

Jobless people left Gate City in droves as they traveled elsewhere to seek employment. My parents were no exception. They left me and my siblings with my paternal grandparents in South Carolina and went to Detroit, Michigan, to work in one of the many plants that manufactured products to support the war effort. However, the pace of Detroit was too fast for my parents, so they returned to Gate City some months later.

My father's frustrations with being unable to support his family began to take a physical and emotional toll. He drank heavily and often was absent from our household for days at a time. I knew little about what he did for a living. All I knew was that he was in and out of our lives, and that he was undependable. Finally, he left my mother, and she began raising five children alone.

My mother had an eighth grade education and worked low-paying jobs such as a custodian and a housekeeper to make ends meet. At times, we relied on welfare to survive. It was during that time that the poverty that plagued society in which I lived began to affect me directly because of the lack of decent medical care. As I mentioned earlier, Scott County had few physicians. This meant that those who did have practices in the area served many clients, most of whom were poor. Because of the poverty, the doctors made very little money. Many of these professionals had their hands full serving their patients. There was little time for them to keep up with the latest research in health care. At that time, I, my family, nor the doctors knew of the disease that was lurking within my bloodstream.

The first pain episode that I can recall occurred when I was four years old. I was walking with my mother along a county road in Gate City on a lovely spring day. I am not sure where we were going, but I do remember that I loved being with my mother. She was a beautifully pleasant chocolate-brown lady who had the world's most joyous smile. And when she smiled, the sun of my world shone much brighter.

On this day, the trees, which had been asleep during the winter, were starting to bud. Flowers had already bloomed everywhere. A slight breeze was blowing. The road was unpaved, and I was kicking rocks in the dirt. All was well with the world. Or so I thought, until a sharp pain shot through my arm. It felt as if a sharp kitchen knife had pierced my skin and cut to the bone. I began crying as the pain intensified. Even though there was no physical explanation that the eye could see, the pain grew worse, as if I were being jabbed repeatedly with an ice pick. My mother tried to comfort me, but her efforts were to no avail. The pain was too sharp. Frantically, she rushed me to see Dr.

Wallace, whom she hoped could diagnose what ailment was causing such severe pain in a seemingly healthy four-year-old child.

The doctor examined me and found no physical cause for the pain. Exasperated, he suggested that my mother rub liniment on my arm. The lotion-like substance was a medicine that she then applied on my skin to relieve the pain and stiffness. Dr. Wallace told my mother to bring me back should the pain continue. Initially though, the possibility of another doctor visit was out of the question. There simply was no money. However, my long crying spells and the searing pain proved to be unbearable to my mother. Money or no money, I had to go back to the doctor. She somehow scraped together enough money to take me back to Dr. Wallace, who knew nothing about my malady. The fact that I was only one sick black child suffering from its wrath, left little room for time or attention in researching the disease at a local level. Dr. Wallace was the only doctor I ever saw in town. Again, he prescribed liniment.

Two of my mother's brothers began to help the family. One moved in with us, and the other lived across the street. Because of my uncles, we had adequate clothes and coats on our backs, shoes on our feet, food in our stomachs, and at least one gift from Santa Claus at Christmas. Over time, it became obvious that whatever was wrong with me was not going away. My mother worked constantly. She left my sister Linda, who was older than I by eighteen months, in charge of caring for me throughout my pain and illness.

Of all the children within my extended family, I was the most burdensome. I rarely ceased to cry and complained of my legs, arms, and chest hurting. My mother did the best she could under the circumstances. As her money would allow, she took me to the doctor and the prescription was always the same - liniment. My ever-dutiful mother took me home and rubbed me down with the stuff as directed by the doctor. She put my sister in charge of me and went back to work. Never once did the doctor suggest that I should be admitted to a hospital for testing.

My illness, pain, and general confusion about my ailment rendered me a loner. I had no friends or playmates other than my older sister, who was my caretaker. I usually stayed at home unless my sister took me out. Rarely did I play outside or interact with other children, if my sister was not around. I spent many days lying around because I was so tired. Performing household chores was not part of my routine because my mother believed that I was not capable, that if I were to help that I would get sick. My sister Linda managed the house, cooked, and cleaned. She managed the other children, who became her personal army. Linda also managed me, though I was her problem child. I would have been one of her soldiers, but I did not have the strength to volunteer for duty.

One of the worst episodes that I can remember, involved a simultaneous pain in my arms, legs, chest, and back, that lasted twenty-four hours per day, for two solid weeks. The pain was so intense that I could not walk; someone had to carry me to the one bathroom in the house.

This is how it would be for the next twelve years—a never-ending cycle of pain episodes, doctor visits, liniment applications, and gradual easing of pain. Word of my ailment traveled around the community, but mostly in whispers about the strange illness that little Judy Gray had. Some folks even believed it was a type of curse.

In between the pain episodes, I learned to read and play the piano, which for a time made me feel happy and like a normal child. One of the most difficult aspects of my illness was that my mother and other folks were not able to see anything outwardly wrong with me. I had no obvious disability, such as a broken bone, walking with a limp or even paralysis. No one could see what I was feeling. I received no concessions if I was ill. If I was not in pain, then I went to school and everyone expected me to perform well academically. If I was in pain, my mother believed it was probably not bad enough to keep me at home. Simply put, my mother accepted no excuses for not attending school. She forced me to go to school whether I was sick or not. My mother went to work as a custodian at a bank at five o'clock in the morning and returned home four hours later. If she found me at home still in bed, she spanked me. She thought I was playing hooky from school. The unfair punishment that my mother directed towards me made me more upset than I already was.

The doctor's reassurance that I would be all right unfortunately reinforced my mother's method of discipline. The doctor told her over and over to rub liniment on me, and that it would help the pain to eventually wear off. My mother took everything he said as the spoken truth. After all, he was the trained, knowledgeable professional.

Over the years, I grew increasingly isolated, knowing I was different from most children. I believe that talking to others about how I was feeling was futile, because no one understood what I was experiencing. Venturing far from home and the security of family to go out and play was out of the question. I was either tired or hurting, or I feared having a pain episode while away from home.

My body was tired, and I often felt pain, but this ailment did not affect the sharpness of my mind. I felt that the wheels inside my head were spinning far beyond my immediate surroundings. I spent much of my time wondering what would become of me and pondering what was out there on the other side of the mountains that might one day change my life for the better.

Meanwhile, Linda, my older sister and caretaker, was more than a surrogate mother. She became a role model. She was gregarious, a natural comedian, and a friend magnet. Linda was the consummate social butterfly. In comparison to me, she was my alter ego, while I lived, trapped in a permanent cocoon, seemingly never to morph into a vibrant, happy, pain-free individual. Yet I yearned to take flight in the world.

As I advanced into my teens, I decided I had to stop feeling sorry for myself and try my level best to overcome my sickness. I crossed the state line into Tennessee to go to high school. I wanted to become a majorette, just like Linda. So I did. Concentrating on that goal did wonders for my psyche, taking my mind off my intermittent pain. I did not worry about my malady because if I did experience an episode, Linda was always right there to help me out. I participated in sporting events and parades, which I loved. The trouble with that was, those activities caused me to spend my entire day's allotment of a valuable currency - my energy. With nothing but fatigue left in my tank, I went home and crashed my head onto my bed.

What I did not know then was that the cold fall and winter weather would be a precursor to the pain. I tried to ignore my illness, and I pushed myself to new heights trying to be a normal young person. Just as Linda did, I took on odd jobs to earn spending money for myself. I washed dishes for fifty cents, babysat, and performed light housekeeping. However, these jobs were temporary and whether I could do them or not depended, of course, on whether I was having a pain episode.

It was at the age of fifteen that I made an important decision. I told my mother I wanted to leave home. My mother showed obvious relief. She had done all she could do for me and could do no more. My Aunt Amanda, who lived in Corpus Christi, Texas, agreed to take me in. When my time to leave approached, my Aunt Ruth in Barnwell, South Carolina, had just died. The plan was for me to meet my Aunt Amanda in South Carolina at the funeral and return to Corpus Christi with her. My rendezvous with Aunt Amanda would prove fortuitous. The next chapter of my life would provide a badly needed answer to the riddle that was my health.

Chapter 3
A New Beginning

"Change your thoughts and you change your world."

Norman Vincent Peale

In the summer of 1958, my mother agreed that I would leave Gate City, Virginia and go to live with my Aunt Amanda in Corpus Christi, Texas. While in Barnwell, South Carolina, I met and became friendly with other teenagers. For the first time in my life, I had friends of my own; I no longer needed to ride my sister's coattails when it came to having a social life.

My new acquaintances were boys and girls between the ages of sixteen and eighteen, who lived in strict, church-attending, God-fearing households. Parents raised children to uphold their own reputations in the community. The words a typical adult most wanted to hear from a child were yes ma'am, no ma'am, yes sir; no sir; may I, please and thank you.

Because I made new friends while I was in Barnwell for my aunt's funeral, I wanted badly to live there instead of Corpus Christi. A girlfriend who lived a couple of doors down joined me in asking my grandmother if I could stay and finish high school there. My grandmother listened to the request, talked it over with my grandfather, and they gratefully agreed. My grandparents' decision was influenced partly by the fact that my girlfriend's parents were well regarded in the community. Staying on my best behavior also helped.

I quickly learned that living with my grandparents was light-years away from the household in which I grew up in Gate City. My grandfather was the breadwinner while my grandmother was the homemaker. He owned an auto repair business and served many customers who regarded him as a first-class mechanic and businessman. As a result, my grandparents had money and prestige, although they were not fantastically wealthy.

As I watched how my grandparents handled their successful business, I could not help but be mystified. These were the parents of my father, who I rarely saw display such responsible behavior in my old household in Virginia. My father proved that the apple sometimes falls *miles* from the tree. This did not matter much to me because my grandfather took on the role of my father.

Living in Barnwell provided me with serious social cachet. I was the granddaughter of Harry Gray, a pillar of the community. My new friends viewed me as well-to-do, and my grandfather made sure I lived up to my reputation. He provided for all of my needs—shoes, clothing, and food—and even some luxuries, such as books, games, and even a bicycle, which I rode only after my chores were completed. I did not ride every day, and pedaling did make me tired. However, I did not complain, lest my bike be taken away.

I was in seventh heaven when I started school in the fall as an eleventh grader. At age sixteen, I had more new friends than I could count. Many of my classmates held down part-time jobs, such as picking cotton, housekeeping, or babysitting. They made their own money, and I too wanted my own cash. Because of my lurking pain and overall tiredness, I rarely did any household chores, let alone hold a job. Still, I begged my grandparents to allow me to work part-time somewhere.

My grandparents were well aware of pain episodes I suffered during past visits and were unsure about giving their permission. I persisted in asking to work until my grandfather reluctantly allowed me to try my hand in the cotton fields. And guess what? I lasted on that job all of one-half day. Seeing an earthworm slither through the soil between the cotton plants was enough to make me quit. Creepy, crawly things such as worms or insects scare me to this day. I would have gone home at that moment, but no one was available to give me a ride. After I asked to try something else, my grandfather allowed me to work as a domestic for a white neighbor whose home was within walking distance.

When I arrived at the house, I entered via the side door, as was customary for black housekeepers who entered white homes. The lady whom I worked for had prepared a sandwich and a drink for me and put it in the refrigerator until lunchtime. I cleaned and ironed all day for a whopping two dollars and a half. That was good money for a day's work and today is equal to approximately twenty dollars. I did well when compared to other kids who made only two dollars a day.

While walking home at day's end, I witnessed a darker side of life in South Carolina. I was in a region where white racism towards black people was abundant and mean. Whites riding in cars threw objects at blacks walking along the road, which frightened the heck out of me. Whites especially harassed black individuals who walked while drunk. I learned that racism was more open and prevalent in South Carolina than in Gate City, where the societal divisions were more about rich versus poor than black versus white.

No one threw anything at me during my walk home that day. At that point, I decided to quit the domestic job if I had to go there on foot. I never again asked to work outside the home. To ensure that I would never be a target of racists, my grandparents kept me off the streets.

At age sixteen, I traveled to Jacksonville, Florida, to spend the summer with my Aunt Louise, whose husband managed the local swimming pool and who got me a job there. As fate would have it, pain struck again. Normally this would be a bad thing, but there was a positive aspect to this pain episode—my suffering pain in Florida led me to finally learn what had been ailing me for so many years of my young life.

Aunt Louise contacted her physician, Dr. Washington, and described to him my symptoms. The doctor had her bring me in for tests. Dr. Washington provided Aunt Louise a diagnosis: sickle cell anemia. This was the first time someone used a name to refer to my pain occurrences. The doctor ordered a blood transfusion and all of a sudden, I felt like a new person. I was ready to take on the world; the pain was gone. Next, Dr. Washington talked to my aunt but not to me.

When we returned home, I waited for Aunt Louise to say something, anything, but she never did. I figured that whatever I had was something I did not need to know about. No adult ever discussed sickle cell anemia with me. It felt like a grown-up thing, and the mindset was not to talk to children about anything of substance. Through bits and pieces of conversations that I overheard, I learned that sickle cell anemia could be fatal, which scared me. I tried not to listen to or read anything about it because I did not want to know that I could die prematurely. If the adults were trying to protect me from this knowledge, then I would just remain ignorant of those details of my illness. Consequently, I never discussed sickle cell anemia with anyone.

Because I was a curious young woman, I often wondered, from an early age, what would become of me and if I would ever be able to live pain-free. As badly as I wanted answers, I decided against asking my elders. Hearing little to nothing about the disease over the years only solidified a growing belief within that perhaps the doctor erred in my diagnosis. Or, I thought, because I was still alive, maybe I did not have the fatal disease after all. Sickle cell anemia, which was later called sickle cell disease, for me was primarily an out-of-sight, out-of-mind sort of phenomenon—that is, until I had a pain episode, which came every one to two years during most of my life.

In between pain events, I lived life as normally as I could. What I did not know was that the sickle cell anemia was causing constant fatigue for me. I would not realize this connection until I was well into my fifties. But as a teenager, I never met anyone with a similar illness. In my mind, that made me different. I learned quickly that life must go on.

At the end of the summer, I left Florida and I traveled back to Barnwell, leaving the pain episode, doctor visit, and diagnosis in Florida. Strangely, I do not remember becoming sick often while living in Barnwell, but when I did, my grandmother took me to Dr. Dixon, an African American physician who lived up the street.

From then on, I concentrated on completing high school. During my junior year, I took classes in shorthand and typing. I was so good in both subjects that teachers called on me to share my expertise with the seniors. I developed a keen interest in business, and one of my teachers expected me to go on to college to pursue that discipline.

My grandparents also expected me to attend college. They decided I would enroll at South Carolina State College, the alma mater of three of my aunts, in nearby Orangeburg. My older brother, who had also lived with my grandparents a few years earlier, graduated from Claflin College, next door to South Carolina State.

Until that time, I never dreamed I would follow my aunts and brother in pursuit of higher education. If I stayed in Gate City, college would likely have never entered my mind. In Gate City, life was about survival.

After graduating high school at age seventeen, I entered South Carolina State in 1960. I never did major in business. Looking back, I believe it was poor career counseling, or a lack of counseling, that shunted me into the field of elementary education, an area that many African American females occupied at that time.

Once again, I became a loner in college. It was a reminder of my life in Gate City. Most of my time I spent in the dormitory room completely exhausted. I only went out to class and to the cafeteria for meals. Rarely did I participate in extracurricular activities. Just like my family in Gate City, my fellow students thought I was lazy. I missed my big sister, Linda. In college she was not there to watch over me. I talked to no one, and my fatigue was just another part of my life that I kept to myself.

I would have strived for an "A" average, but I was always too exhausted to give class lectures my undivided attention. I did just enough schoolwork to get by and that was my objective. I spent many nights lying on my stomach, leaning over the edge of my bed, reading my notes or textbooks, which I'd place on the floor. While some kids studied with friends, or groups and some visited the library, this was my preferred study method.

On rare occasions during those four years, I ventured to the student center to mingle with people whom I met in the dorm. I went to one football game, became tired, and I left at halftime. I never even watched one basketball game.

I do remember having a boyfriend, but the relationship was short-lived because I was always too tired to spend any time with him. I was hardly sociable, so this guy found another girlfriend. I felt sad at the time. However, I felt that there was nothing that I could do to improve the situation. I had grown accustomed to the isolation in my life.

For many people, college ranks as among the best and most memorable years of their lives. This was not the case for me, but I did not complain. I was fortunate to be in college at all. My long-term goals were to earn a degree and get a job. My grandfather paid a pretty penny to cover my first year's tuition payment, so I had to take my education seriously and not play around.

All the while, my sickle cell anemia was lurking in the background, ready to spring into action with no notice. I knew it was a matter of time before a pain episode made an unwanted visit. I was right. When one did occur, I called my Aunt Louise in Jacksonville, Florida, who in turn contacted the campus infirmary and explained what was going on with me. Aunt Louise asked her Alpha Kappa Alpha sorority sisters on campus to help me and ensure that I got to the infirmary, where I received another blood transfusion.

After three wonderful years in South Carolina, life, as it often does, took a turn for the worse. In August 1961, just before I was to start my sophomore year at college, my grandfather died of kidney disease and heart-related problems. I was devastated, as was the rest of the family. The emotional and financial impact was far reaching. His long-thriving auto repair business died along with him because there was no one to step in and run it.

The money stopped flowing and my family's wealth dried up. To finish school, I had to take out loans from the bank where my mother worked as a custodian. During the summers, I went to Jacksonville, Florida, or New York City to work and make money to help cover my tuition and other necessities such as clothes.

Those remaining years at South Carolina State were relatively uneventful, except for a few days in 1963, when my stubborn tiredness lifted long enough for me to go to jail for participating in a civil rights march. South Carolina State served as a safe oasis for African American college students. Every now and then, however, students who ventured off campus, found the surrounding town of Orangeburg to be a jungle of racial hostility. Blacks were harassed, spat upon, denied service in stores, and sometimes even arrested on trumped-up charges.

The few white shop owners who were very glad to take our money still treated us as social lepers. We could buy food, but could not even think about sitting at the lunch counter. We had to eat outside. Resentment built a strong base. When Dr. Martin Luther King, Jr. came to Orangeburg, we eagerly signed on to march on the city. He led the protest against the injustices and indignities that we had endured. Hundreds marched. Then the authorities ordered the troops to turn on the water hoses and direct them at those who were marching in the front of the line. The strong water pressure did not stop the crowd. It forged on. I was one of many arrested.

First, we filled the local jail. The others went to an open field where they stayed until midnight when the buses arrived to take them elsewhere. Men went on some buses and women on others. I was in the group that went to the open field. Our destination was a women's prison in nearby Columbia. For a moment, uppermost in my mind was, "What would my family think of this?" My grandfather, the family breadwinner, had died nearly two years earlier, and I was scrimping to go to school. Did I really have the time for this?

Then I snapped back to reality, and said to myself, "Hell yes, you do. You have to do this for oppressed people, not just in the American South but around the world!" When we arrived at the prison, they took our fingerprints and ordered us to sign some blank papers. I refused to sign, as did three other women.

The angry jailers decided to deal with us, the quartet of insolent black women, the only way they knew how, by throwing us into

27

solitary confinement. After the first night, I awakened to see the general inmate population pass by my tiny window. I called out from my cell and asked why they were imprisoned. The answers came one by one: murder, assault, burglary. I was shocked. I never knew anyone who killed another person. Now here I was, a sheltered little girl from the hills of southwest Virginia, sharing the same space with criminals and learning a hard lesson about life in the 1960s South.

My cell was dark except for a small ribbon of daylight that shone through a tiny window. Light also came in through a slot in the door at mealtime along with something masquerading as food for human consumption. I ate breakfast, which consisted of light bread and syrup. The other stuff in bowls shoved through the door looked like worms. I did not eat it, but I later thought that it could have been ground beef.

They released me from solitary confinement after four days, and I spent another three days among the general prison population. By this time, the National Association for the Advancement of Colored People (NAACP) posted our bail and we went free. The NAACP took us back to campus. We then boycotted the stores in Orangeburg, whose black community trekked to Columbia to shop.

A year after my adventure in civil disobedience, I graduated on time from South Carolina State with a Bachelor of Arts Degree in Elementary Education. Even though I did not pursue my preferred course of study, which was business, I was jubilant that I had reached such a crucial milestone. What I didn't know at the time was just how big of a role that sickle cell disease would continue to play in my life.

Chapter Four
The Vow – In Sickness and In Health

"What a strange distance there is between ill people and well ones."

Winifred Holtby

Mignon McLaughlin said, "A successful marriage requires falling in love many times, always with the same person." This was unfortunately not my experience and had I been married for long enough I would have perhaps succeeded. I did learn a lot from this experience, however, and when I look back now, I am grateful that it made me the strong and independent woman that I am now.

I met my husband at a social gathering in Richmond, Virginia when I was twenty-three years old. He grew up in Lynchburg, Virginia, the only child of doting parents who were in their forties when he was born. His father was a Baptist minister, his mother was a homemaker, and he was close to an elderly aunt and uncle who lived a couple of doors down.

My boyfriend was well-mannered, fun loving, and a jokester. He knew how to treat a woman with common courtesy by opening doors and pulling out chairs for seating. As a wine connoisseur, he taught me how to sip gracefully whenever we dined out. He preferred movies, house parties, and card games as opposed to some of my preferences which included expensive outings such as going to dinner every once in a while.

As the son of a minister, he regularly attended church on Sundays and was involved with its youth programs. His weekly routine would include going to church on a Sunday and usually without me, as this was the one day of the week when I managed to get some rest and recharge after a full week at work.

Armed with both his Bachelor's and Master's degrees in Chemistry, he had all the trappings of bachelorhood: an apartment, furniture, clothing, and a car. Real estate investment was one of his favorite topics. This was long before buying income-generating properties became popular via late-night infomercials. He would definitely be a decent husband and a good provider. He was what folks like to call a good catch. After we dated for five years, he finally proposed and he gave me a very nice engagement ring.

We were married in a big church wedding in Gate City in May 1971. Nearly two hundred guests attended the service. The reception menu included a succulent pig with an apple in its mouth as the centerpiece. We received tons of gifts, but unfortunately we could not afford a honeymoon as I would have wanted. We then moved to Richmond to live in a duplex that he purchased before our wedding.

I was extremely happy to be a wife, but my elation came second to my constant fatigue. For most new brides there are whirlwinds of activity, settling into a new routine with a husband, setting up a new home, and ensuring things are in order, but this was not the case for me. I had to budget my energy, most of which would be spent on my school teaching job.

As we settled into married life we developed a routine in our household where we both knew what our duties were in our home. My husband was an adequate provider and worked consistently as a tobacco company chemist. He loved to cook and entertain guests at our home. I tried to do my best to keep up, baking bread, cakes, and pies. Our events totally drained me to the point where I would not get out of bed the next day. Married life was an exhausting business and I wondered if I could cope.

My husband loved to travel and with him behind the wheel, we hopped into the car at vacation time and drove as far as time would allow us. We once traveled from Richmond to Gate City to visit my family, then to Kentucky to see friends. We then visited friends in Indiana and Nebraska then crossed into South Dakota before turning around and heading back home. On another trip, we drove to Corpus Christi, Texas to see my relatives. As a side trip, we ventured into Matamoros, Mexico, across the border from Brownsville, Texas. There were other, shorter trips, but I gradually ran out of steam and felt too sluggish to travel.

I do not recall at what point he learned I had sickle cell anemia, which by this time was my life's background noise. I do remember my husband visiting me in the hospital, so he knew there was something wrong. I experienced the usual pain and suffering, and I think sometimes he viewed my illness as something that came and went, like a common cold. I felt the same way, thinking it would just go away permanently. But that was not my reality. After a pain event passed, I would get out of the hospital, return to my usual activities, and we would both forget all about the episode for a while.

Over time, my husband became increasingly dissatisfied with his chosen career. He found that he no longer wanted to be a chemist, so he decided to enroll in law school with the hope of transferring to a more lucrative field. After a year, I think he discovered that the coursework of a law curriculum was simply too rigorous and he dropped out.

After a while our relationship changed and there was a lot of stress on both sides; he was doing the best he could to cope with an unsatisfactory career, and I was trying to cope with being married as best I could.

Unfortunately, our relationship deteriorated. Due to my illness, my husband was the primary care giver for our new baby daughter Loree, who was born in May 1974. I can only imagine what it must have been for him taking on the role of a househusband to a spouse too tired to handle homemaking duties. My illness must have had a profound impact on my marriage. He took on a job as a security guard at the local state prison. I think he must have viewed this as a transition back into chemistry from his failed law school experience. He left the prison job after a year to take a position at the local wastewater treatment plant as a chemist.

The impact of all the changes, the frustration and anger and perhaps even fear spilled over on me and our daughter. Needless to say our relationship suffered and our divorce became final in August

1976, more than a year after we separated. Divorce is always an unpleasant experience and I learned the hard way to be more careful when it came to financial arrangements. I received several thousand dollars based on what the courts determined was my share of the properties. We did not retain the properties. We ended up selling. In the end, neither of us realized a profit from our investments.

I had to create an environment where I was able to support myself as a single parent. When I look back now, the blessing I got from this experience was to obtain a true sense of independence. I learned finally to truly depend on myself and to ensure that I had the reserves required for not only my future but for my daughter's future as well.

Effectively, she too became a very independent and self-sufficient young woman.

Raising a child alone was another challenge in my life, in addition to the recurring pain of sickle cell disease. I needed an escape. Since I already held a Master's degree from Virginia State University, I decided to enroll at Virginia Tech to study for a doctorate but I only got as far as finishing the coursework. Writing the dissertation was another matter; I simply did not have the stamina and the discipline.

So then, I decided I would move out of Virginia as an escape from the overwhelming stress of child support issues. I found a college teaching job in North Dakota, of all places. However, I stayed only six months because of my concerns about possible negative health impacts of the cold Upper Midwestern climate. This apparently was not a well-thought-out plan. I returned to Virginia Tech to try to finish my dissertation but still was not successful. It was now time to get serious about finding a job and settling down. Therefore, I returned to Richmond and lived with a friend until I could get back on my feet.

An interesting fact is that when people hear about a potential split, the first thing they say is, "You all need to sit down and talk." It is not that easy; verbal communication is one of the most difficult things in a marriage, especially when things start going wrong.

I have since decided to reflect back on the good things about my marriage, and the biggest blessing I got was my baby Loree. A mother could not ask for anything more. She has been my pride and my joy and has far exceeded all the expectations I had for her. With regard to everything else, I learned through this experience how to be independent and really take care of myself. I found ways to conserve my energy so that when I was with my daughter I could give her my full, undivided attention. I also found a way to empower my daughter to value her education and to be responsible for herself at a very early age.

I learned the importance of communication in relationships; somewhere in my marriage, my husband and I failed to talk and discuss the issues that really mattered. If we had sat down and developed a plan of action to deal with the challenges at hand—my chronic health issues coupled with the arrival of a new baby—perhaps we would have found a way to work things out. It all looks so clear now when I reflect in retrospect, but at the time I just couldn't see the wood from the trees.

All up, the biggest gift I got from my marriage would be the love of my life, my dearest daughter Loree.

Chapter 5
No Excuses!

"If you want children to keep their feet on the ground,
put some responsibility on their shoulders."

Abigail Van Buren

The memory of marching for civil rights in Orangeburg stays with me today, as does my admiration for Dr. Martin Luther King, Jr. and the civil rights movement. To me, this was an act of importance. Growing up in Gate City, I viewed my mobility - economic, social or otherwise - as limited.

Once I moved from Gate City and saw how others lived, I began to see possibilities for myself. Later, I saw that I could fully participate in American life, with a good job, the right to vote, and the right to live where I desired, as long as my pocketbook approved. Dr. King's movement solidified in my mind the idea that African Americans were just as deserving of the fruits of America as anyone else. My marching reflected my enlightened thinking. The status quo, a longstanding system that relegated black people to second- class citizen status, was now on life support, and I would help pull the plug.

I decided I would honor Dr. King's legacy by taking with the utmost seriousness life's most demanding job - raising a human being from birth into a productive adult member of the society that Dr. King and his legions of followers changed for the better. This I did with my daughter Loree. As I came to know Loree during her formative years, I discovered a child who was smart, focused, and independent. My job was to employ my hard-won experience, knowledge, and wisdom to channel Loree's traits into a positive direction. After all, one could say there are criminals who also are smart, focused, and independent. I moved heaven and earth to ensure Loree would stay on the straight and narrow path to success and away from the superhighway to hell.

I cannot discuss raising Loree without first mentioning a person who was like a sister to me, and to whom I owe a great debt. Without my dear friend Pat, I don't know where my daughter and I would be today. I met Pat about forty years ago when we were both enrolled at Virginia State College (University). She was a senior finishing her bachelor's degree in Special Education. I was in graduate school, completing my master's degree in Special Education. I lived on campus at the time, which I enjoyed because of the camaraderie that I developed with people from different walks of life. In our little group, there was Pat (the black girl from Richmond), Laura (a white girl from New Jersey), a girl from India, one from Japan, and one from Korea (but I forgot their names). We immensely enjoyed each other's company and got to know one another's cultures, usually over meals consisting of our respective native cuisines.

Pat and I hit it off right from the beginning. She is a petite woman with a take-charge personality and a heart of gold. I knew her whole family. They adopted me and my daughter as a part of their own. I had no problem calling up Pat and asking if they were cooking for the day. During holidays, I often found myself putting my feet under the table of her mother's house or hers. Over time, Pat looked at me as a big sister. My recurring pain and fatigue did not in any way color our friendship as I kept to my custom of keeping silent on that subject. Nevertheless, whenever pain struck, Pat was always there to provide emotional support. No matter where I was, she would be thinking she had to go see about me. Pat would eventually be my guardian angel, much like my sister, Linda, was in Gate City.

Dominating our conversations was the topic of money and how to get it (legally). We consistently cast about for ways other than traditional employment to increase our cash flows and bank accounts. Pat and I concluded that our chosen paths of teaching would not lead us to financial independence. Why did we choose teaching? Frankly, during that time, that career path was all that we were exposed to as African American women in the late 1960s and early 1970s. In addition, I recall my plan to major in business at South Carolina State was derailed. It would be much later in life that we realized we could do other things.

One way of making money, we decided, was direct selling. We tried marketing Mary Kay Cosmetics, to which I recruited Pat as a member of my down line. Alas, I could not keep up with the demands of selling makeup, lotion, and foundation while motivating down line sales representatives to do likewise. In network marketing, the adage goes, the speed of the leader determines the speed of the group. How true. I slowed to a halt and so did my unit, including Pat. She and I believe we would have been driving the organization's signature pink Cadillac, then reserved for top sales reps, had we stayed with the business.

Our children were born thirteen months apart, Loree in 1974 and Pat's daughter, Nikki, in 1975. Neither Pat nor I intended to become single parents, but those were the cards we were dealt. Now we had to roll up our sleeves and play our hands in the poker game called life. We'd be doing a lot of calling and raising of stakes as we grew into our roles as moms.

Loree and Nikki grew up like sisters, and Pat was always there to do things with them when I was too tired. Pat often had the girls active. They went to the movies, amusement parks, libraries, and other places that kids like.

For a time, Pat and I went our separate ways. With the strains of a divorce, raising a child alone, and generally not knowing how I was going to make it financially, I escaped to school, taking refuge at Virginia Tech to work on my doctorate - or so I told others. I surprised myself by completing the coursework, but I could not complete the dissertation.

I thoroughly enjoyed my position on the other side of the desk, meaning I did not have to prepare lesson plans or assume responsibility for others' learning, as I did as a classroom teacher. I worked in the university's political science department as a graduate assistant, setting up meetings, conferences, and performing other support tasks for professors. Whenever I had to go to the hospital for treatment, my daughter stayed with the head of the department and his family. When it became clear that I could not complete my dissertation, I started to focus on where I wanted my daughter educated. After that brief trek to North Dakota, I seriously looked at the school system in Richmond, Virginia, which appeared to be making a lot of progress academically. I desired to place Loree in a multi-ethnic school system.

We headed back to Richmond. Once there, we moved in with Pat and Nikki, until I could find a place for Loree and me. The arrangement was fantastic, with Pat and me babysitting for each other whenever one of us wanted an evening out. Under no circumstances would we invite gentlemen callers to the place. We kept our personal and social lives separate from the girls.

All the while, my tiredness was not going away, and I felt as if I could not give Loree the proper attention. When Loree was in second grade, I decided to send her to a close family member for school. I thought, "this worked for me when I was growing up, so why not now?" Living with relatives away from me did not work for Loree. She was miserable, and so was I. At the end of the school year, I retrieved her and was determined that I was just going to have to try something different. After giving the public schools four years (including kindergarten) to educate my child, I sought a private school education. Pat moved to another school district in which to enroll Nikki.

Loree was a miracle on two levels. One is that she is even here. The other is that she is free of the sickle cell disease and trait, which are hereditary. When I was pregnant, it did not sink in for me right away that I could be bringing someone into the world with the same illness or who could give the illness to her own child. When my husband and I decided to have a child, we talked to a counselor at the sickle cell clinic at the Medical College of Virginia in Richmond who told us about the risks of having children and passing down sickle cell disease. This meeting marked the first time I learned that sickle cell disease was hereditary. I think I was half-listening. It seemed like the counselor was talking about someone else, not us. That risk really did not sink in for me until five months into my pregnancy.

I underwent weekly testing while carrying the baby. They included blood and urine tests. The physician must have seen something because he sat me down and said I might want to abort. Remember, abortion was a risky procedure, but so was bringing a baby into the world. In the end, thank God, I chose to have my baby.

I had to bring a jug of my urine to the doctor every week for testing until I was hospitalized for three weeks before giving birth. The hospital staff monitored me during that period until Loree arrived by Caesarean section. I continue to be thankful she carries neither sickle cell disease nor the trait.

As I said, Loree was thirteen months old when my ex-husband left us and saddled me with a myriad of issues such as child support, custody, and visitation as well as making certain she received the proper schooling down the road. At one point I was so overwhelmed by it all that I sat and cried until I came to my senses and realized crying releases stress, but would not solve any of my problems. All self-pity would do is keep me locked in a cage.

My limited energy reserves forced me to maintain a plan "B" in the wings. Quitting was not an option, so I continued to soldier on. I adopted a parenting style of doing what was necessary and not dwelling on justifications as to why not. I wanted my daughter to learn that same lesson, that there was no room for excuses in this life.

Loree liked to mimic me. This made me happy. When Loree was a preschooler, we went to dinner at a Chinese restaurant and were seated in a booth with very cushy seats. I plopped down and crossed my legs. I looked under the table and saw that Loree had crossed her legs as well, which had me smiling.

However, I was concerned that Loree would see me come home from work and go straight to bed, and that she would do the same. Fortunately, that did not happen. I never told my daughter about my persistent fatigue and occasional sickle cell disease-triggered pain episodes. I never knew what to say, so I remained silent.

As I settled into the role of being a mother, I set an overarching goal of preparing Loree for a career, rather than a job. In my view, careers make a difference in the world. A job maintains the status quo. I believed in the importance of Loree being stimulated intellectually. She bubbled with curiosity and loved to travel. I encouraged her to share with me every educational experience, her school activities, and descriptions of her field trips.

Managing my daughter, my energy, and my relatively meager finances from day to day took a toll. I welcomed holidays as a time to catch up on my rest. Those breaks, especially during Thanksgiving, were stressful on another level in that I was too broke and tired to go out and buy all the fixings necessary for a complete dinner, so we either dined at someone else's home, or I sent Loree on a trip if the chance arose. Loree usually went to my mother's house during Christmas, which meant she could spend time playing with relatives her age, doing movies, libraries, and other kid activities. That my funds were low meant Loree got few gifts from me.

I wanted Loree to take lessons in a foreign language before she entered kindergarten, but I let someone talk me out of that idea. To my everlasting regret, I put this person's opinion in front of my own, and I gave credibility to the opinion that I was being too pushy a parent by wanting my daughter to speak a foreign language. Not all was lost, however. By the time she entered kindergarten, Loree had a solid foundation in reading, writing, and arithmetic.

Loree attended public schools from kindergarten to the third grade. Over time, I had become increasingly disenchanted with the public school system and its limited view of the purpose of education. I decided Loree needed an education that would prepare her to compete globally, as opposed to learning just enough to enable her to jockey for position with others here in the United States seeking "well-paying jobs."

I often went to the school to discuss the curriculum. I wanted to ensure what Loree was learning was challenging to her and developing her critical thinking skills.

However, as a result of my advocacy, the public school took it upon itself to place Loree in a "gifted and talented" class a couple of hours a day, apparently to get me out of their hair. I was unimpressed. The school could not understand that I was not advocating that my daughter be placed in any type of special program.

I set out to find an alternative educational setting, which more than likely would be a private school, knowing full well such a learning environment would cost me money I simply didn't have. At one school I visited, in 1983, I witnessed students using computers, learning foreign languages, studying maps, and generally working hard on their academics.

Eureka! I had found Loree's new school. It charged students (by extension, their parents or guardians) sky-high tuition. Undaunted, this teacher with barely two nickels to rub together submitted an admissions application to this institution. All Loree had to do to win entry was to undergo an aptitude test. That Loree passed was no surprise to me. She had done her job. Figuring out how to pay the expensive tuition was my job.

Loree was offered a spot in the next class, and I went to work on working the system. For the first two years, after scholarships, Loree's great-aunt paid the tuition. Thereafter, I was on my own. A partial scholarship from the school and my own scrimping covered the rest. I had fun shopping for her school clothes. When she entered school, she looked like she was prepared to do her job. She took to the school like an eagle to the sky and excelled academically.

I raided Loree's book bag once she went to bed at night looking for information to help me understand my daughter. I wanted to know how she approached her schoolwork. I learned she was extremely organized. She created "to do" lists and checked off each completed item. In our conversations, I learned that she thrived from learning new things.

I recall the times Loree sat on my bed and excitedly told me about her daily activities as I lay there on my stomach with my eyes closed, exhausted. I may have looked zoned out, but in reality, I was hanging on her every word, thinking, "Yes!"

Misbehavior by other students irritated Loree because she found that it disrupted her concentration. Fortunately, such shenanigans were rare since the private school only had to make a single telephone call home. Parents understood that their children needed to shape up because the school would not tolerate misbehaviors.

Many of Loree's classmates had a year of French under their belts when she entered. It did not take long for her to catch up. She was soon among the top three students in French. She would later receive a top award for excelling in Japanese and French at her high school graduation exercise. Whenever she came home with information about an upcoming trip, I realized I would have to attend a meeting for the parents. I listened intently. I needed to know the level of educational enrichment the trip would provide Loree, how much it would cost, and of course, how I would pay for it.

I never discussed money in front of Loree when it came to trips or schooling. I called the school's headmaster the next day to determine if scholarships were available for the trips. There were, but like tuition, the scholarships only covered part of the bill. The other portion came out of my pocket. By the time Loree was in the middle school grades, I was drowning in a sea of bills. I thought about placing Loree back into the public schools due to the costs of the private school. I sent Loree on a daylong visit to the local public middle school to see if she wanted to go there. When she got home, she said, in no uncertain terms, "Absolutely not." She witnessed a teacher repeatedly disciplining disruptive students, which she said would interfere with her learning.

The thought of incurring the continued expense of private school overwhelmed me. Yet, I thought, there were other families I knew who were struggling financially. My thinking was if they could do it, so could I. Somehow I had to make this work. When Loree was eleven, I signed her up for babysitting classes. As she cared for two children during her first job, I sat by the phone in case Loree called with questions. Babysitting marked Loree's first foray into the world of work, which lifted some of the financial burden off me. She was able to buy her own toiletries and have her own spending money. Over time, Loree landed part-time jobs in a grocery store and children's retail store, which she held through her high school graduation. There were times I had to ask her for money to cover the utility bill, and she willingly contributed.

Loree was doing quite well both in school and in volunteering in the community. In middle school, she volunteered in a low-income neighborhood, teaching adults old enough to be her grandparents how to read and how to use computers.

Because I made it a habit to live below my income, my clothes were often shabby. Buying shoes for Loree was a challenge because her feet kept growing. As Loree got older, however, my job as a single mom eased. At age sixteen, she got her driver's license, and I purchased her first car with money I saved. I could have jumped for joy. I bought her an old, straight-shift Volvo. She learned how to change gears in the parking lot of our apartment building. I remember praying every time she got behind the wheel that she would safely get to where she was going and would shift the gears correctly. No longer did I need to transport her around town. Now, Loree was able to run errands for me.

During her high school years, Loree took several trips overseas, to France, the Netherlands, the United Kingdom, and even Australia. She also traveled to Canada and Mexico. Within the United States, she traveled to Cambridge, Massachusetts to participate in the Model United Nations at Harvard University. I loved how she would report to me about her adventures abroad. Her stories were so vivid that I felt as if I had been to those same places. She would later travel to the Cayman Islands, Hawaii, and the Caribbean island of St. Lucia.

Private schools stage annual fundraising drives, and Loree's was no exception. Some parents simply whipped out their checkbooks and, well, wrote checks for large amounts of money. I did not have those kinds of funds. However, that did not stop me from searching for ways to contribute. One day, I spied an item in the local newspaper announcing a dinner roll baking contest. I entered, and every day I prepared different types of yeast rolls that I believed the contest judges would find tasty. I encouraged my neighbors to stop by and taste my rolls. I remember agonizing over the brands of butter and flour I would use. Finally, based on my neighbors' opinions, I settled upon the recipe I would enter.

When it comes to serving food, as in most pursuits, presentation is everything. When I submitted my baked rolls to the newspaper, I made a huge splash. I donned a chef's hat, apron, and wheeled in my arrangement on a three-tiered glass table. On the first tier was a colorful napkin as the tablecloth and a small replica of a place setting. The second tier had my rolls covered with a decorative towel.

I made my entrance into the newspaper offices to the Patti LaBelle song "On My Own" being played from a boom box brought by a friend. I moved in a very seductive manner. My entrance caused heads to turn among the employees working on the newspaper's first floor. However, the actual judges never saw my grand arrival since they were already assembled upstairs waiting for each contestant.

It mattered not that the judges missed my entrance. What counted was their opinion of the taste and texture of my dinner rolls, which they judged as winning first place in the competition. When it came time to participate in Loree's school fundraiser, I advertised my award winning dinner rolls as my contribution, and sold out the day before the fundraiser. I could not bake the rolls fast enough. Suffice it to say, my unorthodox contribution was a success. My experience shows that the old cliché, "where there's a will, there's a way," is so very true.

While Loree was a great daughter, an excellent student, and a huge source of assistance to me, she reminded me she was also still human. I found out she had an eating disorder. She had been seeing a therapist in school and the therapist had given Loree a deadline for telling me. When she did not, the therapist called me. We agreed that Loree needed to check into a hospital.

I was devastated. How in the world was I going to pay for this? I never hesitated to provide Loree the treatment because there was a clear need. Loree's father was nowhere around, providing neither moral nor financial support.

After she graduated high school, she deferred her acceptance to Syracuse University for a year. She had originally planned to go to Spain for a year through the American Field Service program, but her history with the eating disorder prompted the program to reject her as too much of a medical risk.

Instead, Loree decided to participate in a program in Massachusetts called Dynamy, which would provide her with real-life work experience and a break from academics. The work experience she chose was with a social service agency. Whenever they had some activity in the community, Loree was right there. She excelled in that program as well, receiving awards at the end of the year. Once she enrolled at Syracuse, she attacked college life with gusto. She took on student loans and scholarships, including the prestigious Remembrance scholarship in honor of the students killed in the terrorist bombing of a Pan Am jet over Lockerbie, Scotland.

I regret missing that awards ceremony because I was in the midst of a sickle cell pain crisis. Wouldn't you just know her father attended the awards ceremony with his chest stuck out with pride? Still, I was glad he showed up because I knew it would mean a lot to Loree for someone to be there for her.

She also, at one point, served as a resident advisor. Loree earned her bachelor's degree in child and family studies in three and a half years. She would go on to complete her master's and doctoral degrees, both in marriage and family therapy, at Syracuse as well. Whenever I visited Syracuse, Loree took great joy in showing me around the campus.

Today, Pat and I both couldn't be prouder of our girls, who were influenced by the choices we made for them as children. My daughter is now Dr. Loree Anitra Johnson, who owns a private family therapy practice in Los Angeles, Santa Clarita and Hermosa Beach, California. Loree likes to travel around on a motorcycle she calls Purple Reign, a nod to *Purple Rain*, the movie and album featuring the artist Prince.

Nikki, a singer, actress, and dancer, performed in the 2010 national Broadway tour of *Dreamgirls*. Nikki is also a nationally recognized health and fitness expert and chief executive officer (CEO) of her own fitness company, Get Fit with Nik, and is often sought after for appearances by the major television networks.

I continue to say thank you to The Collegiate Schools and to Syracuse University for educating my daughter. To Pat, I say thanks for being my other Linda, and to you, Dr. King, I offer my deepest appreciation.

Chapter Six
My Family

"Family is not an important thing. It's everything."
Michael J. Fox

"I hope that my daughter grows up empowered and doesn't define herself by the way she looks but by qualities that make her a intelligent, strong, and responsible woman."
Isaiah Mustafa

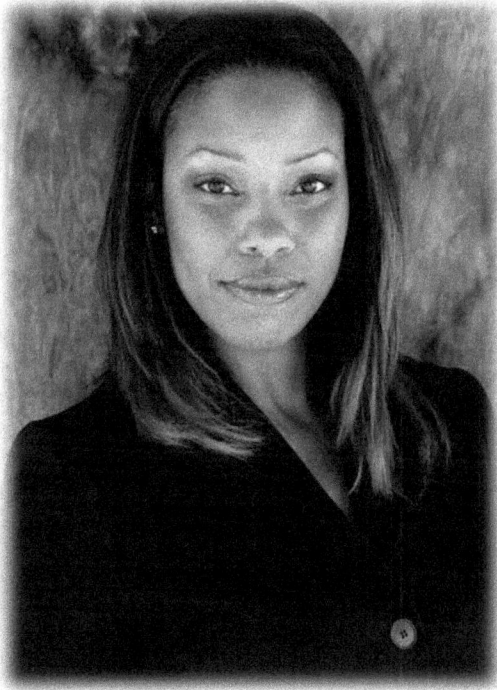

My daughter, Dr. Loree Anitra Johnson

"We never know the love of a parent till we become parents ourselves."

Henry Ward Beecher

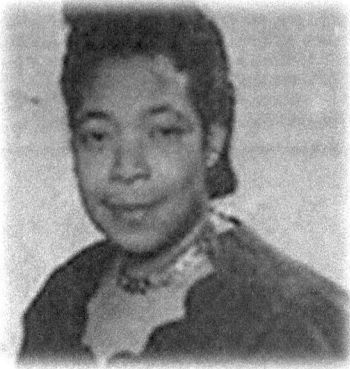

My mother, Janie Turner Gray

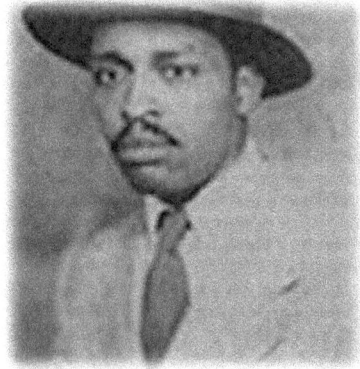

My father, Therman Gray Sr.

"I sought my soul, but my soul I could not see. I sought my God, but my God eluded me. I sought my brother and I found all three."

Author Unknown

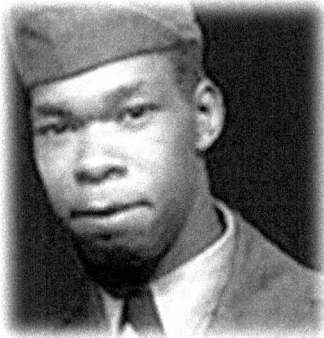

My brother, Donald Wayne Turner

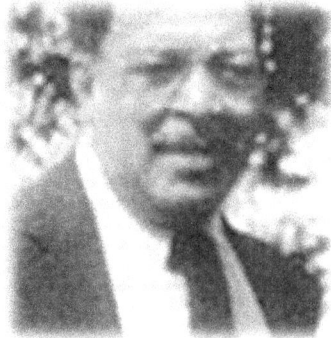

My brother, Therman Gray, Jr.

"You may be as different as the sun and the moon, but the same blood flows through both your hearts. You need her, as she needs you."

George R.R. Martin

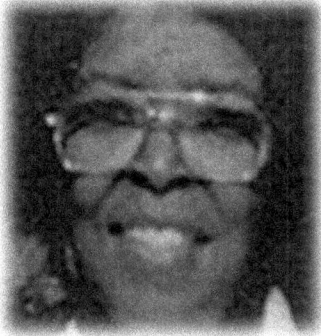

My sister, Linda Gray Lyons

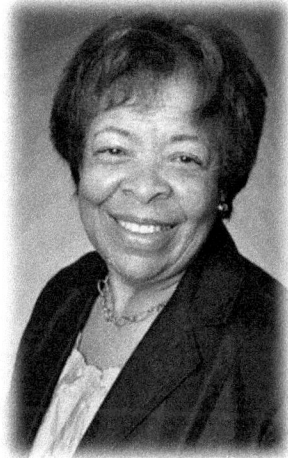

My sister, Dr. Rosemary Gray

'The history of our grandparents is remembered not with rose petals but in the laughter and tears of their children and their children's children. It is into us that the lives of grandparents have gone. It is in us that their history becomes a future."

Charles and Ann Morse

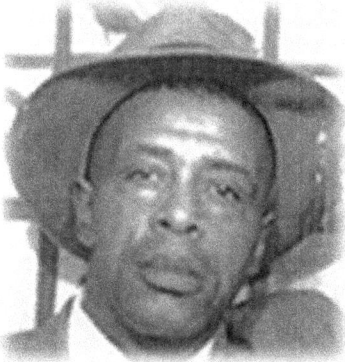

My grandfather, Harry Gray

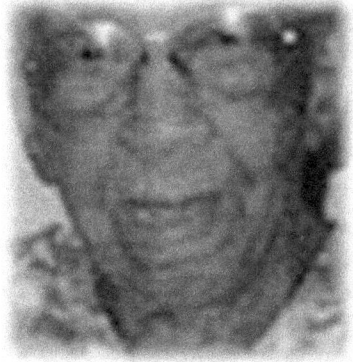

My grandmother, Lula Rountree Gray

Judy Gray Johnson

"Only an aunt can give hugs like a mother, can keep secrets like a sister, and share love like a friend."

Author Unknown

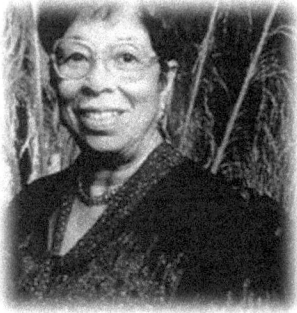

My aunt, Amanda Gray Perry

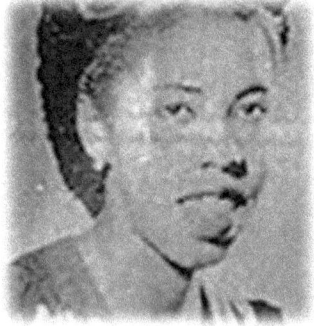

My aunt, Ruth Gray Matthews

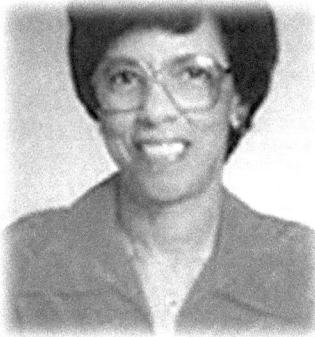

My aunt, Louise Gray Guinyard

"I owe much thanks to my uncles for always being there for me throughout the years. It was great to know that I always had someone I could depend on. You have no idea how much that meant to me."

Judy Gray Johnson

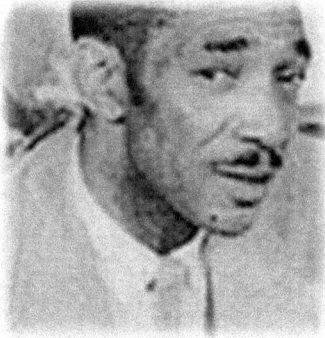

My uncle, Paul Turner

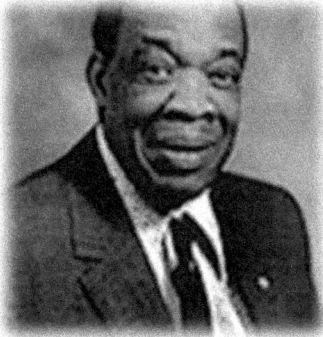

My uncle, Eldridge Turner

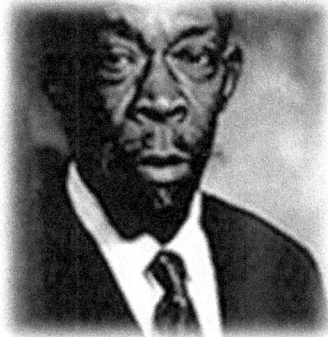

My uncle, Hoyate Turner

Chapter Seven
That "Cushy" Chair

"Don't limit yourself. Many people limit themselves to what they think they can do. You can go as far as your mind lets you. What you believe, remember, you can achieve."

Mary Kay Ash

My family and friends see me as a successful individual. I was once asked, what has influenced me most in my life? I immediately responded, "Sickle cell disease." It is not something that comes and goes or that you acquire later in life. You cannot push it aside and say, "I will deal with that later." It is demanding and relentless. It will make you drop everything you are doing so that you have to deal with it at the moment it arises.

Contemplating the world of work often brings back painful childhood memories. While my sister cared for me, as a surrogate mother, I was extremely aware of my surroundings. On occasion, when someone else was at home with me, I saw my sister go out and make money to buy her own clothes. I watched as my mother and others in our close-knit community went to work in order to bring home money that would take care of their immediate needs. As most people at that time dismissed me as too sickly to do anything, I was keeping a watchful eye on them and learning the ways of survival in this world. People were often mistaken about me. Everyone I knew misunderstood my illness during those days, including me. It felt as though no one believed that I had a brain. To them, I was sickly, and that's all that mattered.

This treatment affected me a great deal. I became observant and reflective. I literally had no one to talk to about my aches and pains, my feelings, or my thoughts and concerns. There was no one there to listen, to whom I could ask questions, or to tell me what was wrong.

This is what it meant for me to be in survival mode. If I were going to live or die, it would be at my hands, and no one else's. It was at a young age that I learned to look for windows of opportunity.

When I was feeling okay, I would get up early in the morning and accompany my mother to work. When I heard that there was a lady that was paying someone to wash her dishes, I jumped at the chance and got the job. I remember thinking, how odd it was that one could earn money for this simple chore. I thought back to how my sister Linda would clean our kitchen, and I attempted to do it the same way. This lady paid me fifty cents an hour and I was overjoyed. My pocket was heavy with money that I had made myself, and I could do with it as I saw fit. I bought myself some clothes, just like my sister. When I got sick, I would have to stop working in order to deal with my bout of illness.

Other jobs that I tackled were babysitting and light housework during the summer. For a while, I lived on the premises of the people for whom I worked. I do not know how I survived, but I did. I was forever fearful that the family for whom I worked would discover that I was an imposter, and that I did not know how to clean house or do anything meaningful at all. I did not tell them that in my house, I was the one whom others cared for, and that I had a serious health concern. At the end of that summer, I had earned quite a bit of money with which I bought many clothes for myself. While there were daily painful episodes, I was able to suck it up and keep going. I just did not talk about it.

As I began my professional career, I had no idea what the future would hold. I had recently graduated from South Carolina State College in Orangeburg, South Carolina, with a Bachelor's of Science degree in Elementary Education. I was anxiety-ridden during my first interview. My main concern was not whether I could do the job but whether I could physically survive and if so, for how long. A school eventually offered me a job for a whopping salary of $4,000 a year, based on my ability to play the piano with one finger.

I loved that school and the community. We each had something to give the other. The staff was warm and caring, and often provided for student needs beyond the classroom. Afterschool projects included the shoe patrol, coat patrol, and other community service projects designed to appeal to student's intellectual curiosity about the world beyond school. This was my first job, and I bought my first car with my earned income, a used Ford.

Child abuse and teacher impropriety were unheard of in those days. It was nothing for teachers to put as many kids in their cars after school and dash off to the city for an evening of fun at the Virginia State Fair or to pick up a group of kids on a Saturday for a day at the museum. It simply meant that if we picked them up, it was our responsibility to safely deliver them home. We would head home around nine o'clock at night. As I dropped each child off, the meaning of a long country road became quite clear; their houses were not close together.

Parents accorded teachers a level of respect befitting royalty. They were eternally grateful for the love, interest, and guidance shown toward their children. As a teacher, parents and administrators respected me and allowed me to do what I had learned to do. I never once heard a parent come to school whining about what they did not have or what they could not afford. As a gesture of love and admiration, they would often pick vegetables from their gardens and leave them inside our unlocked cars during the day. We never knew which parent did what. We did know that this was the community's way of saying thank you, we love you and be well.

No one ever knew, until now, what that groundswell of love and support meant to me. The more the community gave, the more inspired I became to do more. Although for me to do more physically was a detriment to my overall well-being because I did not know how to pace myself. I was regularly exhausted, but I never complained. I looked around at others and saw how they handled their jobs. We were doing the same thing; each pulling our own weight. Yet our recuperation time was much different. All most people needed was a quick nap, and they were raring to go. For me, in my personal life, I was exhausted or completely devastated. I would lie around all day in my bedclothes, and I rarely did housework. My self-image of laziness that I learned as a child was embedded in my day-to-day existence. Although I would often joke about it in an attempt to just brush it off within myself, I began to experience serious self-doubt. The laziness factor was so present on my mind that I began to feel lazy. I do not recall ever going to the doctor about this because it seemed silly to ask for a treatment for laziness. Therefore, I remained silent. It would be many years before doctors would associate fatigue with sickle cell disease. In the meantime, there was only silence about the disease. I continued to undergo bouts of sickle cell crises. I'd head to the hospital and be released, seemingly good as new after receiving a blood transfusion, IV fluids, oxygen and some type of pain killer, most likely morphine. I took no medications between hospital visits. I just went on with my life until the next crisis.

Much later in life, I learned that doctors' knowledge of sickle cell disease was also limited. When I did get the nerve to discuss my fatigue with the doctors, they wanted to give me valium or some other pills that would provide relief.

Somehow I struggled through the school year while using up my sick days. After one year, I transferred to another school district. This was probably the worst professional decision I made. I was not unhappy at my first school, and I could not have asked for a better supportive climate for what ailed me. In the end, it was the money that motivated my decision to leave. The other district paid me an increase of five hundred dollars per year, which increased my salary to $4,500 per year.

Things took a turn for the worse. More often than not, I found myself in and out of the hospital. Doctors routinely kept me in the hospital for at least a week, sometimes two weeks at a time. The unspoken message was to go home and continue with your life until the next crisis. In my mind, I expended my sick days like a drunken sailor spent cash while at port.

While I lost the comfort and security of my first school job, I found a doctor that was gentle, kind, and caring. This was during the racially segregated 1960s, when whites tended to go to white doctors and blacks went to black doctors. I loved my doctor and as I could tell, so did others. If you were to drive by the office of Dr. Charles Sutton on a given morning, you would see a long line of people waiting outside for the doors to open. I spent a fair amount of time in those queues.

It was nothing for us to wait hours to get in to see him. On some occasions, I would wait for five hours to get in to see him face-to-face. Once in, however, you had his undivided attention. Higher-priority medical emergencies would increase the wait times to see Dr. Sutton. I clearly understood that because there were times when I was given priority to see Dr. Sutton because of my painful sickle cell crises. The excruciating pain would command immediate attention. On one occasion, I remember that the pain I felt was atypical of the familiar sickle cell pain episode. Today, remembering that feeling, I may have made my way to the emergency room, but not in those days.

I awakened early that morning with a pain so severe in my fingers that I was unable to make a fist. Because I lived alone, there was no one there to assist me in bathing or putting on my clothes. I could not even hold a washcloth to wash my face. Somehow, I made it to Dr. Sutton's office, and I immediately advanced to the front of the line. He used his stethoscope to poke around briefly and then sent me straight to the hospital, where I stayed for seventeen days after undergoing several evaluations. In the end, the doctors discharged me and told me to take aspirin.

Each hospitalization, and each bout of pain and fatigue that did not require hospitalization, caused me to take time off from work. It did not take me long to use up my sick days year after year. I felt tremendous guilt about missing so many workdays. Whenever I returned from an absence, I sheepishly walked quickly to my classroom. I would try to avoid eye contact with my principal as I passed him in the hallway. I could not figure out what to say to him to make him understand what was going on with me, so I said nothing. This is when I decided to start job-hopping. In my mind, I needed to go somewhere where no one knew me. I thought that changing jobs frequently would somehow help me escape the stigma and the clutches of the infamous sickle cell disease. If I stayed in one place too long, I feared that I would be fired for missing too much work. This prompted me to look for other teaching opportunities, which started a cycle of moving around in an effort at maintaining anonymity.

A nearby school district was looking for kindergarten teachers, and they offered to pay for teacher certification in that area. Since I had an elementary education background, which was a prerequisite for kindergarten education, I met their criteria. They hired me, and I eventually became certified. I worked two years as a kindergarten teacher, which in turn, enhanced my resume.

I often took classes during the semesters to enhance my skills as an educator. At one point, an issue arose that led me into teaching special education. I was teaching fifth grade at the time. Student performance was so low that I was on the verge of failing the whole class. I discussed this with the principal and requested his help in solving this problem.

He agreed to come in and do a demonstration lesson while I sat in the back of the classroom to observe the class as a whole. The picture that emerged was of a class that had many diverse needs. Their needs required more than my skills alone for sufficient remedy in one year. I began attending seminars on children's learning styles. My coursework provided me with diagnostic and evaluation tools, an understanding of diverse learning styles, and the application of teaching strategies that would assist me in meeting the demands of my current class and the future trend in education. It was during that time that my understanding of individual education programs (IEP) emerged.

Information came across my desk that Virginia State College was offering a scholarship with a stipend, for those wishing to pursue a master's degree in special education. After having my transcripts reviewed for acceptance into the program, I discovered I needed only one full year of study in order to complete my credentials for a master's degree in special education. I applied, and they accepted me into the program. This was an easy decision for me because I was not married and had no family obligations at the time.

Armed with a master's degree in special education, another school district offered me the opportunity to develop a high school special education program. Within a couple of years, I moved on to another district to become its director of Title I programs and its elementary programs supervisor. By then, I was going through my very difficult divorce, child custody battles, and child support issues. As a means of escape, I took some time off to work towards a doctoral degree in administration and supervision. The demands of doctoral study were challenging enough, and I was sufficiently attentive to the demands of the coursework, but when it came time to write my dissertation that would eventually provide me with the title of "Doctor," I could not get past the stress of concentrating on the dissertation. That was the end of my foray into higher education.

I gave my career one hundred and ten percent when I was present and not suffering from my disease. The only real problem that I encountered was being able to stay physically on the job. I was always present mentally. I could not understand why I was so tired, and at times, I viewed myself as the most disorganized, alternating with the most organized person in the world. There was always a method to my madness. Instead of writing things down on paper, which sapped the little bit of energy that I had, I kept mental lists. I developed strategic plans of action in my mind, and I carried them out as my energy level would allow.

Despite my sickle cell-related attendance problems, I decided I would do my best to control my reaction to the disease despite my sickle cell-related attendance problems, I decided I would do my best to control my reaction to the disease. I concluded that perhaps others would see me in a new light. The fact that I could work was not in question; but what could I do? I finally realized, to my own chagrin, that I could not pattern my life after those of others. I would have to be more creative. Other people did not have the same obstacles that confronted me. I noticed that whenever I attempted to talk to my friends about it, they quickly dismissed my concerns because they had to get on with their lives. All they could see was someone being lazy. If the pain was bearable, I went to work. After work, I went home and went to bed to rest until the next day. I drove my supervisors crazy by persistently asking about my assignment for the next school year and my room location. I needed to know this before school let out at the end of the year so that I could institute my plan for the coming year. My inquiries made no sense to them, but knowing ahead of time was crucial for me.

Once I learned my room assignment, I mentally planned my approach to setting up for the upcoming school year. Over the summer, I would line up someone to help put my classroom together. We put up background paper (fadeless was better because it could stay up all year), created charts, and gathered supplies that would be needed all during the following year. By the time the other teachers came back from summer vacation, I had reviewed what the mission of the school system was for that year.

The most important thing for me to do was to make sure I did my part in helping the school make progress toward that goal. Whatever the skill emphasized, I was ready, because I was able to focus on this during the summer without interruptions. The secretarial and janitorial staff knew me well, because I was always in the building during odd hours working. The irony here is that some folks viewed me as a hard worker, and some teachers viewed me as an over-achiever as I spent my summers at school. The truth was I needed more time off during the year, but I simply spread out my time over the course of the twelve-month period, rather than the traditional ten months of a teacher contract.

When my pain became unbearable, I had to go in and get my usual *juice*. This meant a blood transfusion, oxygen, IV fluids, and pain medication. When released, I felt like a new person and would race back to work the next day. Some coworkers knew of my illness, but I did not dwell on it. They saw me zipping around the school doing this and that so they just looked at me as if it was a temporary thing while I was in the hospital, as if the hospital had fixed the problem.

Living on a teacher's pay was very challenging. I needed more money. Again, I looked for windows of opportunity. I needed a part-time job that I could perform at my own pace. Whenever it became too much, I redirected my efforts. I sold Mary Kay Cosmetics and Amway products, and I worked as a night custodian and telemarketer of military newspapers. Although I was a good sales person, I had to change course. I answered an advertisement for a night custodian for an office building. All I would have to do is dust, empty the trash, and vacuum. It was a team effort.

Others did the heavy lifting. One problem that I encountered was that I did not know how to vacuum.

The carpet was light colored and I thought it would be simple to run the machine over the carpet, but I had not considered the cord that was attached to the machine. As I vacuumed, I dragged the cord along, unaware that the cord stained the carpet. They had to hire another cleaning crew, and I was out of a job. My last paycheck is somewhere collecting interest because I was so embarrassed that I never went back to pick it up.

Telemarketing, on the other hand, was the perfect job for someone like me. I was able to use my sales skills without having to exert too much physical energy. I soon learned where the most comfortable chair was in the room. The shift change occurred between four o'clock and five o'clock in the afternoon each day. I usually arrived early enough to nab that "cushy" chair. I sat in that chair and rested while I was talking on the phone making sales.

I would get off at eleven o'clock at night. I loved snow days when the districts closed school. If Northern Virginia was snow-socked, it was business as usual in the rest of the country. Therefore, the telemarketing job was always open. On the snow days, at 9:00 a.m., I was at work on the phone dialing for dollars and I was able to rack up some serious money to pay off bills early, build my bank account and allow me the peace of mind that I would not have to ask anyone for money. I often wondered if other employees felt the same way I did. As I observed my surroundings, we were often short of help. People came in when they wanted and too often complained about what they had or did not have. I wanted to scream, "You need to be me for a day." I wanted everyone to know about my serious health issues, my level of education, and the fact that there was no one for me to depend on, but I also wanted to remain anonymous. What I learned from this venture was that having multiple streams of income would be a key to my financial survival.

At another school, the principal suspected there was something wrong, but never asked me directly. He did spend an inordinate amount of time observing me in my classroom to find out whether I was effectively teaching my students. This principal did not hold certification as an administrator, and quite possibly, as a result, he lacked the knowledge, training, and competency to use his time effectively. Rather, he chose to put undue stress on me purely because he viewed my health as a weakness.

He practiced a form of subtle intimidation at a time when employees with chronic illnesses had little recourse other than to take what their bosses dished out, for fear of losing a job. This was long before the Americans with Disabilities Act was enacted in 1991. In part, the act mandated that employers provide reasonable accommodations for people with disabilities and chronic illnesses. But even then, had people known that I had sickle cell disease, they would likely have dismissed it as no big deal. Sickle cell disease was not considered a chronic illness. In fact, it was hardly considered at all.

Once the ADA was passed, I attempted to obtain special accommodations in one school district. However, I believed the application, which required a physician to answer questions about a disabled employee's condition, was inappropriate for sickle cell patients.

The questions:
1. Please describe the nature of the employee's medical condition.

2. How would you characterize this medical condition: mild, moderate, or severe?

3. List the major activities of daily living that are limited by this employee's medical condition.

The physician answered the first question by stating sickle cell disease causes occasional painful crises. This is true, but it did not tell the whole story. The response did not speak to the exhaustion and diminished bodily functions that occur in between crises; I do not know if the doctor was aware of this. The doctor failed to mention that sickle cell disease does not begin and end with a crisis, but that it is a lifelong condition and causes problems that the average person cannot see or understand.

In response to the second question, the doctor characterized my condition as mild to moderate. Once again, the physician provided only a piece of the puzzle. My condition may be mild to moderate at any non-crisis moment. During a crisis, however, the accurate characterization of my condition is severe. The doctor's responses to this application did little to improve my conditions at work.

In response to the third question, the physician listed "none." Again, that was only part of the story. There is nothing that I *cannot* do within reason. I know not to over-exert myself. If I become tired, I know to find the nearest chair. However, it is important for me to make that determination. It is also important for employers to understand that that's just the way it is.

I understand now that it was rare then to find someone who fully understood the extent of the disease. I should have asked someone who understood sickle cell disease to complete the form so that the answers would adequately address my needs. For this reason, due to the physician's inability to satisfactorily respond to my needs, the school district denied my application for ADA accommodations.

I always tried my best not to draw attention to myself. However, the most egregious incidents stand out in my memory. One day, at the end of school, a crisis began in my leg. Somehow, I was able to get the message to the principal. She came down to my room and escorted me up to the teacher's lounge. Not once did she reach out to assist me in any way. I had to hobble along unassisted in excruciating pain. It was not until I got to the teachers' lounge that someone called an ambulance. This particular crisis resulted in an eight-day hospital stay. I laid flat on my back receiving oxygen, IV fluids, and morphine every four hours. There was no attempt to wean me off any medication or to help me get my strength back before discharge. I did not even walk myself to the bathroom and back. I remained flat on my back.

Suddenly, on the eighth day, at about eight o'clock at night, the doctor came in and abruptly told me I had to leave because the insurance companies would no longer pay for my treatment. Since I arrived at the hospital in an ambulance, my car was still at school. Sometime during the week, a colleague drove my car to the hospital so I would have a way home, once released. Still under the influence of narcotics, I fumbled around in the parking lot to locate my vehicle and then drove myself twenty miles to my home.

When I moved on to another school, I never told the principal that I had sickle cell disease. Someone I knew from my past had told him. If he had any concerns about the disease's impact on my ability to do my job, he should have approached me to schedule a meeting. That never happened. I went into the hospital twice while at this school. The first hospitalization was due to a crisis. The second was because my dosages of medicine needed adjusting.

Despite my hospitalizations and absences, the principal still never discussed the issue with me. His solution was to remove me from the classroom. Henceforth, I covered for other teachers. I would like to believe that if the school board knew how he handled my situation, they would have dismissed him immediately.

My substantial salary and level of education attested to my professionalism. Yet he placed me in a position as a floating teacher, without a class of my own and without children to teach. This went on for a few months that year. I did not feel I could approach the principal with my concerns for fear of coming across as weak or different in a way he would not understand. Therefore, I said nothing, and he said nothing.

Later I joined a special education curriculum, where I shadowed a small number of students but received no guidance in the form of expectations for the students or me. Then I taught a health class consisting of two grade levels. Initially, I taught both grade levels in the same classroom. Later I was required to teach one of the grade levels in a classroom on a different floor. Throughout this experience, I often wondered why the administration believed I was qualified to teach health.

During the summer, I requested special accommodations for the following school year: a location near a bathroom and unlimited access to water. I never knew that such an innocent request could have created such a firestorm. The principal, upon hearing the news, apparently went berserk. He was involved in several telephone conversations between his office and the district's office of equity and compliance regarding my accommodations. He apparently did not like the situation and made no secret of his displeasure.

My accommodations consisted of a room near a restroom and near a water fountain. I was allowed to have unlimited water in my room. This apparently was too much for the person in charge of making teacher classroom assignments, who was one of my fellow teachers. When I called to see where my room would be, she took it upon herself to "dress me down." She said she was tired of people calling the school asking for this and that on my behalf. She insinuated that it appeared as if she was not doing her job. "Miss so-and-so has been here over nine years and does not have any special accommodations. I don't know why you have to have any!" she said to me.

I called the teachers' union to complain that there was a breach of confidentiality, and that the principal had revealed personal information with someone who was not my supervisor. A union representative agreed to go with me to see the principal, but I decided to wait and hear from equity and compliance about any regulations governing privacy. Equity and compliance agreed to come to my school the following day and agreed to talk to me then. I gave the representative my phone number but never heard from her. I called her office several times after that, but she returned none of my calls. I gave up because it seemed that the whole issue was part of a larger problem beyond me.

Despite the fact that while I was given a classroom near a bathroom and had unlimited access to water in my classroom, I drank less and less water. The reason for this was that students cannot be alone in a classroom, and the administration never found the time to send someone by my room to monitor my class while I used the bathroom. Therefore, I just had to hold it.

Many school districts lack special accommodations for the disabled. I personally applaud those that do. However, I believe school districts should regularly monitor and review the implementation and effectiveness of their disability accommodations policies in schools, not only on paper, and on the premises, but also by surveying and gaining input from their disabled employees.

I worked in one district in which the policy was to complete certain paperwork with the doctor's signature verifying my sickle cell anemia history and additional health concerns. This information went to the principal, stating that I had a disability. No other information, to my knowledge, existed. No one ever interviewed me to ask what I needed in order to be an effective teacher and thus have a successful school year.

While the principal knew that I had a disability, she did not know what the disability was. One day, when I was feeling a lot of discomfort in my legs, I thought I had better talk to my principal, anticipating what might turn out to be a crisis. I told her that I had sickle cell anemia, and that I was feeling some discomfort. In the event that I should have a crisis while at work, I would ask that she would be willing and prepared to handle it quickly. She thanked me for letting her know and asked me to let her know if I needed anything. Fortunately, I was able to finish the day. At home, I took some pain medicine and went to bed. The next day I returned to work. From that moment on, the principal and I never had a substantive conversation about it.

However, she found it necessary to visit my classroom often from that point forward. It often felt as though she lived there. Subsequently, my mid-year evaluation reflected that I could do almost nothing right. As a veteran classroom teacher, with many years of experience and educational training, I knew that I could do something right.

This would become the worst year I had ever had, not just as a teacher, but also as an employee in the general workforce. I was the recipient of unsolicited help in the classroom. Someone would show up at my classroom door unannounced and state that they were there to help me. With little notice or respect for my privacy, space, and personal needs, I felt as though I was being put on the spot to make lightning-quick decisions.

At some point in my teaching career, I took a break from the classroom and ran for president of the teacher's union. This probably was one of the most interesting and challenging jobs that I ever held. I had long been involved in union activities over the years, mainly as a recruiter. When the presidency became available, my nomination appeared. I received input and advice from several folks, including my daughter, who encouraged me to run.

The problem with my supporters was that they did not understand my health issues. In retrospect, if I had understood it myself, I would have used this as a moment to educate others. They deserved to know the unpredictable nature of the disease that might render me unable to perform the responsibilities of president for indiscriminate lengths of time. Conversely, I struggled with how to share information about my limitations without the appearance of whining, making excuses, or being viewed as an invalid.

I sucked it up and ran for office anyway. The good news was that I won; and the bad news was that I won.

Within a week of taking office, I realized that I had made a mistake. I did not know what to do, so I said nothing. The job, because it was new, caused me even more daily exhaustion than teaching, which was something to which I had grown accustomed. The union presidency, by contrast, required me to climb a steep learning curve. I had to familiarize myself with the union contract, and I had to travel around the county school district, interacting with various stakeholders. These stakeholders included members of the county board of supervisors, board of education members, and the union members themselves. So many people sought my attention. They needed me for this or that. They needed their union president.

I carried a bag of tricks in my repertoire to get rest during the day, especially at staff meetings. I would sit away from others at the conference table. This puzzled participants who naturally wanted me to sit closer to them. But what I was doing was trying to prop up my feet on an empty chair under the table with no one noticing.

Union board meetings were generally miserable experiences. I was typically so tired I could not concentrate on the discussion. I always sat in the corner at an angle so I could rest my legs under the table. I was happy when someone did not show up, because the absence gave me more room to maneuver my legs beneath the table.

I found myself anxious to hurry through agendas at meetings. In my mind, I would often beg others to stop the discussion, and stop the bickering because I need to go home. Unfortunately, my fatigue caused me to focus on myself rather than on the union business at hand. I felt tremendous guilt during this process because I felt I could not properly carry out my duties. I steadfastly refused to bring my personal problems into the workplace. To try to explain an illness that no one understands is horrendous. I could only come across as whiny and making excuses for my lack of activities. Of course, what was I going to say to my board members? As the boss, I had to set an example.

Whenever there is a change at the top of any organization, there is frantic movement among members to jockey themselves for various support positions, similar to American politics when the nation's President begins selecting his cabinet. The teachers' union was no exception. I was grateful to have people around me, steeped in integrity, who shared my vision of representing the district's educators. A major focus in my administration was the curriculum. Our belief was that if the curriculum addressed the needs of the children, it would produce better students, thus allowing teachers to do what they were trained to do, which is teach.

Those who were willing to help gave me the opportunity to delegate responsibilities, which is not only a factor of success for someone in a position of power, but was also a necessity for my own personal survival. Others did not know it, but in my mind, I appointed them as presidents of their respective domains.

Being union president meant traveling out of state to various conferences. I hated the exhaustion that this would bring. I flew to Atlanta once without oxygen and it was a disaster. Another time, I was sitting in a hotel lounge at a business meeting when I suddenly became overwhelmed with exhaustion. I abruptly ended the meeting, stating that we would need to continue discussing business in my hotel room.

Thankfully, the attendees declined. I also flew on union business to Las Vegas. I had a crisis and I ended up in the hospital.

Despite the difficulties that I encountered serving as union president, I completed three terms. I ran for a fourth term, but I was defeated. My role as president was to provide for the union, not myself. I was sad for the educators and employees in my office because of the change in leadership, but I was ready for this phase of my life to end. I left office satisfied that I had done everything to the best of my ability to represent the district's educators. It was time for someone else to take over.

While I believed I was enhancing my resume by moving from district to district and pursuing advanced degrees, I never stopped to think how this transience would look to potential employers. As I look back, I am almost certain that my employment history was a roadblock for some administrative positions because no one wanted to take a chance on a teacher who had a history of not staying long in one position. Now that I am retired from public education, I have already started thinking about my next job. I think about waiting tables in a restaurant and developing my writing skills. I have a lot more to say about life and about taking charge of one's self.

Chapter 8
Sickle Cell Survivors Deserve Dignity, Too!

"It does not matter how slowly you go as long as you do not stop."

Confucius

While attending a national convention in Las Vegas in July 2002, I awoke in my hotel room to an impending sickle cell crisis, with pain in both thighs. I took a taxi to a local hospital, arriving at nine o'clock in the morning on July 17. As I filled out the appropriate forms, I told the receptionist that my pain was growing worse.

No one in the emergency room seemed to be in a hurry to treat me or to take steps to make me comfortable. Finally, they beckoned me to an examination room. The escort did not offer me a wheelchair, nor did she attempt to assist me as we walked. I hobbled behind her on a pair of painful thighs. The first nurse on duty came to assist me. I told her I needed to go to the restroom. She pointed across the hall, indicating its location. I stumbled to the restroom with no assistance.

When the doctor arrived, I told him of my history of sickle cell disease and of the pain in my thighs. I also told him my treatment typically consisted of oxygen, fluids, and morphine. I emphasized that the morphine kills the pain and prevents me from having an over-extended stay in the hospital. I also told him I have used a self-pump for administering morphine. The doctor responded that a pump was unavailable but that he could prescribe a morphine injection.

A short time after I received the morphine, the doctor returned and said he had signed papers for my release. The morphine had not yet worn off, and I was still groggy. I don't recall whether I received oxygen while in the hospital. Still, I was extremely upset about my release occurring so soon after taking a powerful pain medication. I was concerned about having to go back out into the Las Vegas heat with little to no fluids administered. The doctor wanted to prescribe pain medication, stating that I could take a cab to have it filled at a nearby pharmacy. When I expressed concern about going out into the heat, his answer was to send in a social worker to talk to me. I was under heavy medication and I was unsure why I needed to talk to a social worker.

The same nurse who saw me earlier walked over to tell me again that my release was imminent. I again told her I needed to use the restroom. She then asked, in a nasty tone, if I wanted to go across the hall or to use a bedpan. I told her I did not think I could make it across the hall. She grabbed a bedpan, slung it up under me, and left the room.

When I began to urinate, I missed the pan, wetting my gown and bed. When the nurse returned, she was furious at finding my gown and bed wet. I guess she was angry that she would have to clean up the mess. She stated, "Sit over there!" I told her I could not because I was wet. She then went off on a tirade. She half wiped the bed down, which would dampen the clean sheet she placed on it. The nurse then threw a clean gown on the bed for me to put on. I told her I needed to wash myself. Her response was to pull a handful of washcloths from a cabinet and throw them toward me.

The nurse then ran the cloths in cold water. When I felt how cold they were, I refused to use the cloths, insisting on cloths dampened in warm water. She grudgingly complied, giving me the warm washcloths before leaving the room. The hospital insisted on releasing me and wanted me to sign the release papers. After such shabby treatment, I refused to sign any papers and hobbled out of the hospital. I returned in a taxi to my hotel room and went to bed.

In between convention sessions, fellow convention-goers would check on me and bring food to my room. My participation in convention activities became very limited, almost non-existent.

I left Las Vegas on July 19. While on the plane, I became sick, prompting the flight attendants onboard to administer three tanks of oxygen. A nurse on the plane checked my vital signs. The airline crew radioed ahead to have paramedics meet me when the aircraft landed at Dulles International Airport in northern Virginia. After seeing the medics, I elected to go home instead of to the hospital.

When I saw my regular doctor a few days later and explained to him what occurred in Las Vegas, he performed the necessary blood work and sent me straight to the hospital for admission. During my four-day hospital stay, I received four units of blood and several units of IV fluid. It turns out I was severely dehydrated.

Las Vegas, an entertainment center and the original mecca of legal gambling in the United States, loves to market itself as a city offering first-rate hospitality to its visitors. I was disappointed that the personnel working at the hospital where I went for treatment did not fulfill that promise. I reported the treatment that I received to the hospital administrator. The findings of their investigation of August 2002 contained the following: (Patient) was given five milligrams of Morphine through an IV and Phenergan, twelve and a half milligrams IV. Notes taken on the case revealed that the investigators reviewed the records and discussed them with the office supervisor. They were unable to prove that the facility provided negligent care. The physician ordered and provided appropriate treatment based on the documentation that he reviewed and the complaints that I expressed at the time of the emergency department (ED) visit. I was unable to seek recourse for the lack of professionalism that I experienced on behalf of the nursing staff. It was suggested that the complainant (me) may want to forward the complaint to a medical examiner's board based on my complaints of inappropriate care by the physician.

After I made repeated complaints to various governmental agencies, they all adopted the same position that the hospital personnel did nothing wrong. Among the organizations to which I wrote in a plea for help were the office of a Nevada United States senator, the National Association for the Advancement of Colored People (NAACP), the Las Vegas Chamber of Commerce, the Better Business Bureau (BBB) of Southern Nevada, and the Nevada Bureau of Licensure and Certification. Of the organizations to which I reached out, I received responses from all but the U.S. Senator.

Over time, I began to believe that most medical professionals regarded my emergency room visits with increased suspicion. The unspoken attitude among medical professionals whom I encountered was that I was an addict seeking a fix. I discussed this with my doctor, who affiliated his practice with my local hospital. He said his experience has been that while working in Philadelphia, he knew very few sickle cell patients who were not addicts. The doctor did acknowledge that I was not an addict, but his assurance did little to make me feel better.

Later I transferred to another medical practice affiliated with the same hospital facility because the original medical practice no longer accepted my group health insurance. I continued to experience suspicion from medical personnel whenever I showed up at the emergency room in excruciating pain. I asked my new doctor to write the emergency room personnel a letter that I could produce on demand that explained my condition. Instead, this physician told me that the next time I visited the emergency room I should request the staff to call him to verify my condition. This was humiliating for me.

The years 2008 and 2009 were particularly difficult. In 2008 alone, the crises seemed to hit me with increasing frequency. That year I had three major episodes that required me to go to the emergency room.

In January 2008, I went to the hospital for a transfusion because my hemoglobin had dropped to dangerous levels. In preparing me for treatment, the nurses connected me to intravenous fluids for the two days I was there. I knew this would cause me frequent urination, so I asked for a bedside toilet or "potty," which would ease the process of relieving myself without having to drag the IV stand back and forth to the bathroom.

The first night was uneventful. But on the second day, I noticed the nurse administered the pain medication hastily, causing me to become nauseated. Usually the pain medication is administered slowly via the IV.

Giving me the medicine so swiftly, it caused such a shock to my system that I rang for the nurses to tell them I was about to vomit. It took five minutes for someone to bring a pan into which I could throw up. The nurse left the pan on my bed, leaving without staying to check on my condition.

I vomited no food but fluid and pain medication, which left the basin half-full of greenish stuff. The basin remained on my bed for several minutes after I buzzed the nurse's station for help. When the nurse finally showed up, she quickly took the pan, emptied it and was about to leave. I had to stop her to ask for a mouth rinse, which she grudgingly provided.

The nurse placed a cup into the bedside toilet to measure my urine. I was told not to place tissue in the cup. I complied. However, no one continuously checked the cup all day to the point that it was full, to the brim, due to my repeated use. Had I used the potty once more, I would have been sitting in my own urine. I called the nurse's station shortly after 6:00 at night to have someone empty the toilet cup. During that interval, I called repeatedly, to no avail. I eventually asked for the nurse supervisor. Amazingly, no one seemed to know her name. At one point I was asked why I wanted to talk to the supervisor. I responded that it was important.

The man I spoke with said the supervisor was in a conference and would see me later. Another time I spoke to a woman. Finally, at seven forty at night, the regular nurse's aide arrived at my bedside, and saw I was quite upset. She said she had emptied my toilet several times that day. I advised her to look in the pan so she could see it was full. She did not look, but she did empty the pan. This aide claimed that no one told her that my toilet needed emptying.

Fortunately, my roommate was a witness to all of this nonsense. As had become customary, I wrote yet another complaint letter to the hospital. *"…I am very upset by this type of treatment. Your staff needs to understand that I was admitted to your hospital several times last year and probably will be again as long as there is a need. Unfortunately, this is the closest hospital, and I do not usually have a choice of facilities. If they are unwilling to give me quality care and to treat me with dignity, then they should find another line of work. I would appreciate someone letting me know that they received my complaint."*

During my second crisis, in March 2008, I went to the hospital by ambulance. As usual, the pain was agonizing and probably was one of the worst episodes I had experienced since childhood. The hospital staff gave me an overdose of morphine. I believe it was the result of benign neglect and sloppy recordkeeping. They gave me ten milligrams of morphine, but apparently it did not do any good because I was still in pain. So within the next two hours, they apparently gave me another ten milligrams. A couple of hours later, I was administered three grams of some other opiate painkiller.

At that point, I had twenty-three milligrams of painkillers running through my system. I apparently exhibited symptoms of someone who had overdosed, and the staff quickly had to find a way to reverse its effect. I remained in the intensive care (telemetry) unit for several days. As I write this, I truly believe I was close to death on that day.

To add the proverbial insult to injury, the crisis came on two days before my daughter and I were to meet in the Cayman Islands for a relative's wedding. By the time my daughter had learned of my condition, I was stable. After having spent more than a combined three thousand dollars for the trip, we decided that she would attend the wedding without me.

There was another crisis and resulting hospital stay in September 2008 that was particularly exasperating. Initially, after receiving a substantial amount of sedatives, I slept a lot due to the medication. When the staff brought me to my room on the floor, I was the only occupant. Later, another patient moved into the room. I did not know the patient, and we never spoke to one another because the curtain remained pulled between us.

What I learned from overhearing her conversations was that she was in her eighties and appeared to be a very sweet person. The last thing I would ever want to do was make her feel bad or uncomfortable. I did not know why she was in the hospital and that was not my concern. However, another problem that she had, that appeared to be unrelated to her hospitalization, was that she was hard of hearing.

This became noticeable to me on a day that I was not requiring much medication and therefore I was much more alert. My roommate turned her television volume all the way up. At first, I said nothing, hoping that someone else would say something. When it became apparent that there would be no change in the decibel level, I summoned the nurse assigned to me. I told her of my discomfort and asked her to say something to the patient. She said she would speak to her supervisor. She came back and said they would be willing to move me to another room. This was unacceptable to me, and I refused. She said there was nothing else she could do. Mind you, neither she nor the supervisor had said anything to the patient. I then requested to speak to the supervisor.

When the supervisor eventually came, I was startled to see how very young she seemed. My concern was that she would not know how to handle the situation diplomatically. I was hoping for a more mature nurse who would tactfully know how to tell this elderly patient that her television was too loud. Instead, she seemed annoyed that I refused to move and immediately went over to the patient and said I was upset about the television being too loud. She then left the room.

There was no change in the sound level. I requested pain medication. When the nurse brought it to me, we again discussed the sound level. She left the room without giving me the medication. I wondered what happened to the medication when she took it back. I did not receive the medication until several hours later, when another nurse came to me that evening. I surmise that they pulled her from another area of the hospital to "deal with me," because the staff was more than annoyed that I was complaining about the noise in my room. I wondered if the needle she used on me was the same as the one brought earlier but never used.

I later asked my new nurse if I could speak to her supervisor. When I explained to the supervisor my problem with my roommate's television volume, she clearly showed frustration. She walked to my roommate and said, "Your roommate does not want to hear the TV." Her tone of voice with the other patient was soft and apologetic. I told the nurse she had misinterpreted what I had said. The nurse turned on her heels and left the room.

My roommate's television volume still had not changed. I rang the buzzer and the nurses on duty took their time answering. The TV was so loud that when the nurses finally answered, they could not hear me speaking. They had to shout through the intercom to ask what I wanted.

A supervisor returned to the room, this time with hands on hips, as if she were going to tell me a thing or two. I told her I wanted to speak to her supervisor and that I needed a form on which to file a written complaint. She said she would get me a complaint form but did not despite my repeated requests. She finally said she did not know where the forms were and that the other supervisor would bring one when he came.

When a clinical technician came to take my vital signs, he, with no prompting from me, asked my roommate to turn down her television, which she did. I told the technician I would list him as a witness to the loudness about which I had been complaining.

The floor supervisor finally came to see me and gave me the complaint form to fill out. After I told him what had happened regarding my roommate's television and that I was planning to report the hospital to any federal agency from which the hospital receives federal funds, he said he would talk to the nurses. He then moved my roommate to another room.

The next morning, my discharge occurred rather abruptly. I told the doctor I had no one to pick me up from the hospital until late afternoon. The nurse told me that checkout was usually at eleven o'clock in the morning, and she would speak to a social worker. They arranged for a cab to take me home. I have to admit this was the fastest discharge I ever experienced from a hospital.

As you can imagine, I was not one of the most popular patients among the emergency room and general hospital staff. Nevertheless, I did not go to the hospital to be liked. I went for treatment. Unfortunately, sickle cell anemia is a very painful disease. To stabilize a sickle cell patient, medical personnel must immediately administer oxygen, intravenous fluids, and administer pain medications through the use of an IV. Until this is done, I am unable to feel relief. Morphine helped me to feel better. Without treatment I would cry uncontrollably, become self-centered, and lose all semblance of dignity. I imagine the disease affects others differently, but there are many similarities for those of us living with sickle cell disease. If you want to know what sickle cell anemia pain feels like, imagine placing your hands flat on a table, and hitting the tips of your fingers with a hammer. The resulting pain radiates throughout the arm for an undetermined length of time. With sickle cell anemia, the radiating pain is constant until the patient receives pain medication.

Eventually, the head of the emergency department finally designated himself as my personal physician for whenever I arrived in the emergency room. In other words, he treats me whenever I come in with crisis symptoms.

It is important to share my experiences with readers because hospitals tend to be seen as pillars of the community. They have a large public relations outreach. However, a hospital is only as good as the treatment they provide. This includes compassion, empathy, and an understanding towards all patients from all members of its staff. In addition, hospitals are rarely held accountable for their errors. Written complaints regarding wrong treatment or poor bedside manners tend to be ignored. The staff adopts the same trained response to any given situation. It seems the only way to get the attention of hospital administrators is to file a lawsuit.

Hiring a lawyer is problematic for many people who generally lack the time and financial resources to do so. Once hired, the lawyer must go up against a team of attorneys who will pull out all stops to defend the hospital. They do not intimidate me at all.

The problem with sickle cell anemia patients seeking redress is due to the limited knowledge of the disease among the legal profession. I consulted with several lawyers regarding the overdose I sustained in 2008. However, even though they agreed that the medical staff was guilty to some degree of malpractice, the lawyers would not agree to represent me because they did not believe my case was worth it to them financially.

They felt that they could win the case, but questioned whether they could get a big enough settlement to cover their expenses and make a profit. Lawyers can understand the impact of a broken arm, the loss of a limb, or the loss of life. Their understanding of mistakes made while treating sickle cell crises, by contrast, is virtually non-existent.

One lawyer agreed to contact the hospital on my behalf to seek an out-of-court settlement. The hospital's letter to the attorney, in essence, said they did everything correctly given my condition; but the resulting complication, while regrettable, did not place my life in jeopardy. The letter also stated they could not substantiate any negligence or inappropriate care on the part of the medical staff. Therefore, the letter concluded, a settlement was not warranted. The questions remain: is it appropriate to give a patient approximately twenty-three milligrams of opiates in less than a six-hour window? And was anyone monitoring the level of dosage administered within that short span?

I lost confidence in the ability of the attorney to handle my case satisfactorily. However, I felt very strongly thinking about this case and the horrible treatment I suffered at the hands of the medical profession. Every day, I looked at the calendar and knew that the statute of limitation of two years to file the case was growing near. I was not intimidated one iota by their hotshot lawyers. I was determined to handle this case myself.

My main concern was my ability to understand the legal jargon necessary to answer the hospital's responses to the complaint. I was aware that they might try tactics in court to delay and to confuse me. However, with that knowledge, I lined up several people with legal knowledge who could explain to me the meanings and use of the various forms that I would need to file in the case.

About twenty-four hours before the statute of limitations was to expire, I called the hospital to determine if they were certain they would not settle. They said they made the right decision. I was close to filing my own lawsuit, but my health was deteriorating and might have prevented me from filing papers with the court by the prescribed deadlines. Therefore, this alone ended my quest for justice.

Hospital records show that during a three-year period, I practically lived in hospitals and doctors' offices with sickle cell-related problems. My concerns continued. I wrote t o the head of the hospital, who in turn passed it along to the director of clinical services for a response. This is my letter:

Dear:

As a Sickle Cell patient complaining of pain in my right thigh, coughing up blood, and pain around my waist (ribs) especially when I coughed, I checked myself into (blank) Hospital Emergency Room around five thirty at night on April 30, 2010.

At triage, they took my vitals and then escorted me to room nine. The doctor treating me was Dr. (blank). After listening to my complaints, he asked what is usually done for me. I told him that they usually give me fluids, oxygen, and blood if my hemoglobin is low enough. He ordered x-rays for my chest, and IV fluids. For pain, I told him that they do not give me Morphine because the hospital overdosed me before.

I am only to be given Dilaudin for pain. In order to give me the fluids and medication, they had to do this through the vein. I told the nurses I was a "hard stick." It took the nurses, doctor, and an intern to finally get a line going into my vein nearly one and a half to two hours. I was stuck several times in both arms to no avail. Finally, the nurses got Dr. (blank). He attempted to go through my neck with a needle twice. When he first looked at it, he said he saw two good veins. The first try did not work. He said he had to go deeper. He put some medication in my neck to help numb the area before he went deeper. He said it worked. He did not wait around to see if it had in fact worked. As soon as he left the room, this effort failed as well. He sent the nurse in to take the needle out of my neck. Eventually an intern came in and stuck the needle in my leg. It worked the first time he tried. They then hooked me up to an IV and gave me one milligram of Dilaudin.

I was then unhooked from the IV while they took me to x-ray. When I returned from x-ray, I was hooked up again to the IV. Later, someone came in and told me my hemoglobin was 8. Later when I was discharged it was written up as an 8.3. I was asked what the pain level was and I told them it was between a five and a six. The only thing they said about my coughing up blood is that x-rays did not show anything.

The nurses started coming in suggesting that I could be going home. I told them that the pain had not sufficiently subsided and that I needed more pain medication. They gave me another .05 gr. Dilaudin. They wanted to know if I had a way to get home. I told them that my car was outside and there was no one to call. I asked if I could stay until the medicine had a chance to wear off or at least for twenty-three hours. That way, they would not have to admit me and it would give the pain a chance to subside. The doctor finally came in at approximately one o'clock in the morning and told me he was discharging me. In other words I was being kicked out. He told me that I should consider outpatient blood transfusion should the pain worsen.

The medical charts can determine the time that medication was given to me. I was allowed to hobble out of the emergency room without anyone seeing to it that I had a safe way home. I got in my car, under the influence of narcotics, and drove myself home.

Because motion causes you to vomit, I had to pull my car over on the road twice to vomit en route home. They gave me no oxygen and did not give me a full bag of fluids. It was obvious that I was very dehydrated due to the difficulty of finding a vein.

Looking back, I wonder if I had been stopped by the police, would they have charged me with driving under the influence. If so, whose fault would it have been? One item that I did not address in my letter was that an intern injected me through the leg while being observed by nurses. I believed that registered nurses did not have the authorization to inject patients in the leg. I have long questioned whether it was legal for an intern to perform the injection. If so, should he have been supervised by a physician? There was not a physician in the room at the time.

Here is their response:

Dear Ms. Johnson:

After receiving your letter today, I am writing this letter to follow-up. We understand your concerns and appreciate you taking the time to bring them to our attention. Patient care is a priority for the Administration and Staff here at (blank) Hospital. We work very hard to ensure that our patients receive excellent medical care and are treated with understanding, respect and kindness.

However, if for some reason we fail to meet your expectations, we appreciate our patients or their family members letting us know. Your concerns are being reviewed with the appropriate hospital management for further action and follow up. In order to address all of your needs and assuring that we are meeting your criteria of excellent service, I would ask that you have your nurse notify the unit director for a one-on-one meeting upon admission to address your needs at that time.

(This implies that I would enter the hospital with a private duty nurse. Also, I am usually in a great deal of pain when entering the hospital. Surely, that would not be the best time to have a conversation with anyone. I believe what they are trying to say is, "Announce yourself upon entering the building!")

We are in the process of yearly competencies and will include IV push reeducation. Thank you for your patience in this matter and for your interest in the quality of service provided by all of us at (blank) Hospital. If you have any questions or concerns in the meantime, please do not hesitate to contact me directly.

We will then provide you with unit management contact information and follow-up with you on a regular basis to assure we are meeting your care needs. The following action items are taking place and will continue to take place. Staffs are receiving service excellence coaching, hourly rounding and huddles to review each individuals care needs and safety needs.

This response was not favorable. It was unacceptable. I then directed my complaint to the Department of Health Professions, which regulates physicians.

I received the following response from an administrator:

Dear Ms. Johnson:

I am writing in regards to your complaint regarding (blank), a licensee of the (blank) Board of Medicine.

The board is authorized to investigate complaints that are lodged against its licensees. The Enforcement Division of the Department of Health Professions conducts investigations for the Board. When an investigation is completed, the Enforcement Division provides the board with an investigative report.

The Board reviews the information in the investigative report to determine if evidence exists to support a violation of the laws or regulations governing the healing arts. If the totality of the evidence appears to support a violation at a clear and convincing level, the Board may pursue a resolution of the matter with the practitioner through one of several statutory options.

Living With Sickle Cell - The Inside Story

I am writing to advise you that the Board of Medicine has completed its review of the investigative report in this matter. Based upon the information available for its thorough review, the Board has determined that it will not initiate disciplinary proceedings.

The Board thanks you for your interest in public safety and protection, and for bringing this matter to the Board's attention.

This response compelled me to take this to the next level, which would be the federal government. What is troubling about this response is that they simply said they will not initiate disciplinary proceedings. Not once did they interview me, nor did they provide me with a copy of their report. Therefore, I was left with the option of accepting whatever they chose to put on paper. To this day, my troubles with emergency rooms and doctors reluctant to treat sickle cell patients continue.

I was admitted in 2010 to the hospital with yet another sickle cell crisis episode. My evaluation by the medical personnel found an acute worsening of my kidney function, likely a result of sickle cell crisis and volume depletion. I was put on intravenous fluids. The doctors and nurses know me to have chronic kidney disease, which is secondary to sickle cell disease, as well as hypertensive nephrosclerosis.

I had trouble breathing to the point where I hyperventilated. They administered oxygen, but I remained in a relative state of unconsciousness. I came to when I was administered a drug called Narcan. I was taken to the intensive care unit for observation.

Again, I was overdosed. A physician's report said I had an episode of over-sedation while in the emergency room and was treated with Narcan. A pulmonary specialist then examined me.

None of the doctors was willing to discuss my condition with me. When the lung doctor came to see me prior to my discharge, I had asked what happened to me. He answered, "You were given too much medication." He promptly left my room before I could question him further. It seemed everyone who treated me was tight-lipped. I wonder if they were afraid of letting something slip that would be grounds for a lawsuit. I believe they were aware of the settlement I demanded relating to the last overdose episode.

Reading this, a person might think I was the cause of this bad medical practice. I am sure that they knew all about my prior difficulties. During one of my visits, one nurse made a point of having me complete an evaluation form, as if to say: we know who you are; we know you like to complain; but please make our lives easier anyway by giving us good reviews.

The daily report asked patients to complete a card each time a nurse did his or her rounds, usually once an hour. The report card asked for hourly rankings of pain, positioning, potty condition, environment, and other. There was a space for the nurse to initial each hour. The rating could be excellent, fair, or unsatisfactory. There was also a space for comments.

Later, a doctor who claimed to be restructuring his practice, asked in a survey for my opinion of the services he rendered. He wanted to know if I would consider staying with his practice should he restructure it in a number of ways.

While visiting this same doctor, he let slip, ever so bluntly, "I hate sickle cell disease! It is not like pneumonia where you can treat it and be done with it. With sickle cell you never know when, where, or how it will occur..." He got no argument from me.

Immediately, I felt his frustration. I so agreed with him. As a doctor, he has been trained to solve problems, provide solutions, and make it better. Where does he turn to for answers? Sickle cell disease is complicated. There are no permanent solutions. Since there is no cure, treatment is often met with uncertainty. I remember thinking as I walked out of his office, he (doctor) can move on to other patients in which much more is known about their ailments. For me, I walked into his office with uncertainty and I left out of his office with uncertainty. There was no escape for me. Like it or not, the effects of sickle cell anemia is always with me, in everything I do.

On one occasion, I phoned the emergency number,

complaining about the onset of a possible sickle cell crisis. The doctor on call said, "You don't sound like you are having a sickle cell crisis." I quickly got off the phone and went back to bed. I tossed and turned for the rest of the night, wondering if I should go to the emergency room before the pain got worse. I ended up waiting until three or four hours later and went to the hospital on my own. I could not let the pain become unbearable otherwise it would be that much longer before I could get relief. I ended up being admitted to the hospital the next day.

Not all of my treatment experiences have been negative. I cite the Medical College of Virginia Hospital in Richmond, Virginia (MCV), as a hospital that is well versed in the treatment of sickle cell disease patients. When I went there for crisis treatment in the 1980s, they knew exactly what to do. I would appear at the intake desk and mention that I was a sickle cell patient. The clerk noticing that I was in extreme pain, immediately swung into action. In short order, a team of medical professionals whisked me into the emergency room, connected me to an IV, administered oxygen, and immediately hooked me up to a morphine pump. This allowed me to self-administer the pain killing medication intravenously. At various intervals they would ask how much pain I was feeling on a scale of one to ten, with ten being the greatest pain. When the pain level dropped between three and four, MCV's staff would ask if I was ready to return home. They never had to admit me for a sickle cell crisis. As a hospital facility, MCV is the yardstick against which I measure all other facilities in their treatment of sickle cell disease.

On two other occasions I found it necessary to be admitted to Georgetown University Hospital (not for sickle cell disease, but for esophageal disticular surgery, and again related to an earlier surgery.) I received such excellent treatment that it was hard for me to believe that I was in a hospital. My experience was so pleasant, I was actually sad to be discharged. I wrote several letters of praise to the staff. Here's one:

Judy Gray Johnson

Dear:

At sixty-seven years of age…, with a chronic illness (Sickle Cell Disease), I have seen more than my fair share of hospitals and emergency room facilities. My experiences have been such that I feel that I am more than qualified to evaluate those medical services administered to the public.

… it was necessary for me to visit your emergency room. I was so pleased with my treatment that I felt compelled to write this letter. As a supervisor, you would have been so proud of your staff. The emergency room was rather busy, and I was amazed at how your nurses handled themselves under duress. Each of them came into my room with a very pleasant disposition and tended to me as necessary. When they had to discuss something privately, they stepped outside of my room and discussed it. I did not have to lie there and listen to someone else's problems. They were very courteous and professional with each other as well.

I hope you place this letter in their personnel file. It should be a reminder of how patients view them and also serve as a database when looking for someone you can turn to when the need arises to train new staff. It is okay to tell them that when I grow up I want to be just like them!

Chapter Nine
Yes, I Have Sickle Cell;
No, I'm Not a Drug Addict!

"We want people to feel with us more than to act for us."

George Eliot

"Tell me, Mrs. Johnson, are you taking any narcotics at home?"

When I heard those words, I experienced a range of emotions, including shock and insult. I could not believe my ears. I was in my late fifties and had been a schoolteacher all of my adult life. To have reached this point, there is no way I would have entertained the idea of using narcotics, e.g. illegal controlled substances, much less actually use them at home. Unfortunately, narcotics are the primary medication that doctors administer when patients are dealing with pain management.

This crisis, like the one I described in the first chapter of this book, is typical of how I am treated as a sickle cell disease patient. The crisis, which led me to be hospitalized from October 26-29, 2002, was one of severe pain and uncontrollable crying. My bed was in a row against the wall of the hospital's emergency room, as were those of other patients.

The doctor never used a stethoscope on me. She came over to me and said the patient next to me was in critical condition and that she would attend to me as soon as she could. The young female physician went back to her station, which I could see because it was directly in front of my bed. I kept crying. She again walked over to me and repeated herself, this time more forcefully, that the patient next to me was in bad shape, and she would get back to me as soon as she could. She then returned to her station and shared a laugh with a nurse.

Apparently, my crying was too much for the emergency room staff. They moved me away from the other patients. I asked repeatedly for the doctor and was told repeatedly she was coming. More than an hour passed before I saw her. When my bed was in front of her station, I never saw her treating any other patient.

Finally, she came back to me, accompanied by a male nurse. Through my shrieks, I told her I was appalled that she would lay another patient's health issues on my shoulders. The physician leaned over me and said, "Mrs. Johnson, that patient was dying. I was appalled that you did not understand." She then asked, "Mrs. Johnson, are you taking any narcotics at home? That's a legitimate medical question."

This doctor's emphasis on the word narcotics, her body language (elbowing the male nurse next to her as if to say to him, "check this out"), and her attitude in general suggested to me that she was insinuating that I was a drug addict. Recent reports document that many sickle cell patients who descend on emergency rooms seeking pain medication are wrongly suspected to be addicts. This young doctor wrongfully added me to that list of suspects. I was angry. Still, the intense pain prompted me to answer her questions to hasten the administration of medication to ease and eliminate the pain. I felt like less than a human being and was on the defensive because I had to convince her that I did not take narcotics at home.

The physician left my bedside. She returned some time later, standing several feet from my bed, as if she did not want to share space with me. She told me I could choose to go home or to be admitted. She threw back her head, wiped her hands as if to say good riddance, turned around, and marched back to her station.

I was admitted and eventually received four pints of blood. I believed this doctor exercised questionable judgment by even offering me the option of going home in my condition.

The incident in that hospital's emergency room left me so angry that I filed a complaint with the hospital administration, which led to a flurry of documents flying back and forth over the next several months between me, the hospital, state health officials, and even the federal Center for Medicare & Medicaid Services (CMS).

My complaint letter was dated November 10, 2002. Less than two weeks later, I met with various high-level administrators at the hospital. I felt like the meeting was a waste of time, because I believed these hospital staff members were patronizing me. One administrator indicated the emergency room doctor inquired about narcotics because they need to know what medications patients are taking. That information, the administrator said, would assist the doctor in providing good medical care and in making sound medical decisions.

I understood all of that, but my complaint centered on the manner in which the physician asked the question, the use of the word narcotics, her body language, as well was what I detected to be some attitude. Her bedside manner, so to speak, was lacking in dealing with me, a patient crying out in extreme pain. I told the hospital staff that I had never in my then fifty-nine years been so rudely questioned by a medical professional.

I later spoke to my primary care physician about the situation, and asked if he would write a letter verifying I was not a drug addict. He said he would be very happy to write a letter to the hospital staff, if necessary, verifying that I was not and never have been a drug addict. However, he never found writing the letter to be necessary.

This was not my only complaint about the hospital's treatment. I experienced adverse treatment only a few months earlier, in July 2002, and during a stay in 1998. What follows, printed verbatim from the report, are the findings of an investigation of my 1998 and 2002 complaints by the hospital and CMS' Center for Quality Health Care Services and Consumer Protection:

Allegation #1: A Medical Facilities Inspector from the Center for Quality Health Care and Consumer Protection conducted an unannounced Medicare/Medicaid complaint investigation of not only my stated Emergency Room experience, but an allegation that during my hospitalization in 1998, I went for four days with no bath, the nursing staff did not provide needed assistance with meals, and that the staff was not sensitive to the needs of patients with sickle cell anemia related to pain.

Findings: After verbalizing my complaints to one administrator on July 8, 1998, a meeting was held to further discuss my concerns with several other administrators. The hospital did not have records of the meeting.

The Center interviewed three current patients who were dealing with pain management. According to their report, there was no problem because the patients appeared neat and well groomed, spoke complimentary of the nursing staff, and was seen and treated in a timely manner. According to their findings, a patient entered the emergency room with abdominal pain, was seen by a physician immediately upon arrival at 13:20, pain medication was ordered at 16:45 and was given at 17:15, thirty minutes later. There are a lot of unknowns here. However, I only wish that my treatment could have been so quick. This is the big question: Why not? Their conclusion is that they were unable to substantiate.

Allegation #2: During my hospitalization from July 22-25, 2002, staff emptied my roommate's bedside commode in the shared bathroom toilet, spilling the contents on the toilet and did not clean it off. One nurse told me that she was "too busy."

Findings: They toured specific medical units, which included occupied and unoccupied patient rooms, clean and dirty utility rooms, kitchen areas and outpatient infusion area. They found that some areas needed cleaning of dust. All of the patient rooms including the bathrooms were clean. The Emergency Department was also toured. There was a series of discussions among the nurses regarding my allegations of unhygienic conditions in my bathroom. The supervisor instructed the patient care technician to thoroughly clean the toilet after each dumping of the roommate's commode. In addition, the roommate was moved to another room that very evening. Conclusion: Staff adequately addressed the concerns at the time the complaint was voiced. Current investigation could not substantiate unhygienic conditions in patient rooms.

Allegation #3: When I went to the Emergency Room October 26, 2002, the physician was not timely and I had to wait in severe pain for over an hour. The physician stated that she and staff were busy tending to a patient who was dying. I felt the physician was unprofessional in telling me information about another patient. I saw the physician talking and laughing with nursing staff while I was still waiting. When the physician asked me "what narcotics I was taking at home?" I felt that question implied I was a drug addict and was inappropriate. Additionally, the physician offered to let me go home or be admitted and told me she would no longer be responsible for me. My pain medication was administered frequently and in small doses. I was not sure the medication was administered properly.

Findings: I arrived at the Emergency Room and signed in at 0945 on October 26, 2002. I was immediately triaged as urgent and taken to a treatment room. I was initially taken to a monitored bed in a bay area just in front of the nursing station. My chief complaint was pain in both legs due to Sickle Cell crisis. The triage nurse wrote, "Pt is yelling in pain, very uncooperative." The treatment nurse's notes read "...upon admission to Rm. #15, pt moaning and yelling." Nursing staff and the doctor attempted to comfort me. I continued yelling, became argumentative non-compliant with staff. This RN heard pt state, "I don't care about anyone else, and you need to take care of me." Their notes showed that I received six milligrams of morphine sulfate IV(intravenous) at 1005, twenty minutes after arriving in the

ED. I received another six milligrams thirty minutes later. The treatment nurse wrote that at a quarter till eleven in the morning I received a second round of medication because I had not had any relief from the first dose. At twenty-five minutes past eleven o'clock, the treatment nurse noted that I was "... far more calm, resp (respirations) quiet, non-labored." Their notes also stated that I was "inquiring re: efficacy/timeliness of efficacy of meds." According to the ED physician's history and physical documentation, at ten forty in the morning, fifty-five minutes after I arrived at the ED, the physician wrote under the section for medications, "I asked pt if she takes any narcotic pain medication at home. 'I don't like the implication that I'm a narcotic addict.' I denied the implication but she continued to argue."

The nurse's notes further showed that I was given six more milligrams of MS04 at eleven thirty in the morning, four milligrams at five thirty in the evening. The physician's clinical impression was "1. Acute Sickle Cell Pain Crisis; 2. HTN; 3. Anemia; 4. Hypomagnesemia." The physician's notes contained the following documentation timed at 10:57 on October 26, 2002:

"Pt brought back to core ED from triage c/o sickle cell pain. She was yelling loudly. We made her aware that there is a critical pt in the ED requiring all of our resources at the moment and that someone would be with her shortly. Pt. stated, 'I don't care about other patients you need to be taking care of me... I should have standing order for pain medicine... look at my records.' Verbal order given for analgesic and at 10:50." She stated that she was 'more comfortable.' At that time I tried to discuss how the ED operates and she became argumentative, 'I don't want to hear it... don't go throwing that in my face.' I left the room to give her some time to settle down and resumed her care from there."

The ED physician noted "after twenty-two milligrams of morphine, pt states that her legs still hurt and that she prefers to be admitted."

Specific staff and I were interviewed separately, along with any formal written complaints made. After requesting a meeting with specific members of the medical staff stated above, a meeting was held with me on November 21, 2002. The hospital did not have written meeting minutes, nor did they generate any correspondence to me following the meeting.

The Center interviewed specific staff members who were in attendance at the meeting on March 13, 2003. The staff member stated that the meeting lasted about one hour and members spent most of the time listening to my concerns. Staff members characterized my complaints as being mainly about the ED physician telling me that there was another critical patient. I stated that this was inappropriate and a breach of patient confidentiality.

The other main point, according to staff, was to express my feelings about being asked by the ED physician if she were taking any narcotics at home. Regardless as to how staff tried to explain it, I was still angry about being asked about narcotic use. It was explained that getting an accurate history of medication use was necessary to best prescribe pain medication that would help her during the crisis. Staff tried to explain that pain medications are often narcotics and there was no intention to suggest that I was addicted to narcotics. I stated that my complaint had more to do with "attitude" than about my medical care.

One doctor, during the meeting, stated that he had reviewed my medical records in preparation for the meeting. Before the meeting ended, the doctor told me that the ED physician was young and may benefit from feedback regarding the complaints against her and that he would speak to the ED physician.

The complaint information is part of the hospital's overall Quality Assurance Process. The grievance policy was reviewed. The policy stated that (an administrator) was responsible for providing feedback to the complainant. However, the policy did not specify that the feedback needed

This investigation added insult to injury. From this experience, I garner that the real conclusion is that patients enter a hospital at their own risk. It to be as specified in the regulation at 42 CFR 482.13 or that the feedback needed to be in writing. Staff stated the (hospital) would make the needed changes to the policy.

Conclusion: Unsubstantiated.

Often it feels as if the health care profession views sickle cell disease, which afflicts predominately African-Americans, as so insignificant that whatever treatment they dole out is good enough.

I escalated my complaints, this time by writing to the hospital's chief executive officer and to the state health commissioner. In my letter, I posed the following questions regarding the hospital's findings:

- Do you support this type of description for a sickle cell patient in crisis?
- What consequences should doctors and nurses face when so characterizing such patients?
- Are you even just a little bit disturbed by the adjectives used to describe my behavior, a patient in crisis?
- Please address the appropriateness of telling a patient as sick as I was about the potential death of a patient in the bed beside me.
- For a sickle cell patient in crisis, please advise as to the correct behavior they should exhibit before the medication has a chance to work.

I further stated that I was insulted and distressed over the conclusions of the final report and wanted to make an appointment to discuss the matter further. The following was the health commissioner's response:

> Your primary concerns did not fall under state licensure or federal Medicare/Medicare regulations that govern hospitals…the Center's investigation revealed no regulatory violations by the hospital in regard to the care provided to you…It is regrettable that the physician was not more sensitive to your needs and presented in a manner that was offensive to you. I hope you will find some satisfaction in knowing that the hospital took your concerns very seriously and addressed them with its staff and the physician.

The hospital's top administrator responded via a surrogate. Her response:

Concern: Timeliness of treatment of pain.

Records from your visit indicate that you arrived and were triaged at 0945 and received your first dose of pain medication at 1005. Twenty minutes for triage, assessment, IV start, and medication administration is within national standards for the timely treatment of an urgent Emergency Department patient.

Concern: Appropriateness of questions about taking narcotic medications at home.

When someone is in severe pain, as you were that day, it is not uncommon to take prescription medication at home for pain relief prior to coming to the hospital for further treatment. In order to prevent a potentially fatal drug interaction or overdose, it is necessary for your providers to know about all medications taken at home. Your concern about the manner in which this question was asked of you was shared with the physician and staff and we apologize for the way you felt.

Concern: Reference made about another patient's status.

As you know, we must take care of the most critically ill patients first in the Emergency Department. Sometimes this means that we cannot address other patient needs as quickly as we would like. We feel it is important to inform patients if there might be delay in their care due to another patient's situation. Although we do not feel that a breach of confidentiality occurred as the patient's name nor a view of the patient was provided, your concerns were shared with the staff and alternatives for handling such a situation in the future were discussed. Our staff needs to be sensitive to this and I feel confident they now are.

Concern: Overall concern about sensitivity and understanding of needs for sickle cell patients.

The (blank) director... has used your feedback as an opportunity to expand the staff's knowledge on care of a patient with sickle cell. Also, she has obtained from Howard University Hospital excellent staff training materials on understanding the needs and issues of sickle cell patients. We believe that our staff will benefit from this training program.

She went on to state "we appreciate the opportunity to respond to your concerns and believe that there will be a positive outcome as a result of our internal inquiry."

Now, mind you, for some inexplicable reason, neither CMS, the state, nor the hospital ever interviewed me. Here is my response to the Center for Quality Health Care Services and Consumer Protection:

This report is filled with lies, distortions, and attempts to discredit me in the worst kind of way. Let's take things in chronological order:

First Paragraph: I requested the address for the Medicare/Medicaid office complaint department from you and you provided me with that information. I wrote them for an application and information about filing a formal complaint, and I never heard from them. Yet the Centers for Medicare and Medicaid conducted an onsite visit, according to your letter. How were they brought into this picture when I had not made a formal complaint with them? It appears as if your office, knowing I was going to contact them, contacted them before I had an opportunity to tell them what I thought were the issues, thus tainting the independent investigation. Please explain your office's relationship with the Center's and in detail, an explanation of the various codes you have cited.

Based upon your stated findings and conclusions, I am delighted that after my three complaints in June/July 1998, July 2002, and October 2002 it appears as if things have gotten better for some patients. However, this does not mean that my earlier reports were inaccurate, and I did not suffer at the hands of inept employees. There is no way that you can interview current patients and employees to determine whether something occurred to me at an earlier time. I note that you reviewed the Hospital Administrative Policies for Patient's Rights and Patient Grievance Process.

Please advise me what it says about the appeals process when there is a clear dispute about what has happened. What recourse does the patient have to ensure that what is reported by the medical facility is the absolute truth?

Allegation #1: I stand by the stated allegation. Does it not cause you to wonder why there were not written records of this meeting? Was I to keep the records? To interview *current* patients who are dealing with pain management in no way has any bearing of what happened to me in 1998. This whole analysis indicates that things have gotten better for other patients as a result of my earlier complaints. You should have interviewed my daughter. She could have told you about the condition she found me in when she flew in to take care of my hygiene.

Allegation #2: I stand by my stated allegation of what happened during the timeframe reported. I cannot address current findings. If the facilities were as described, then again award me a medal for bringing lapses in procedures to supervisory attention. I am protesting very loudly your investigation of this particular complaint...it is presented as a trivial matter and not the serious issue that it was. You did not state what the supervisors found when I initially reported the incident. Did they in fact find a soiled toilet seat? Rather than take responsibility for their own lapses in procedures, they are attempting to place the responsibility on me, the patient, for all of this. Furthermore, it somehow puts the blame on the patient that was moved from my room as if by moving her, the problem was resolved. No, I was not happy with the moving of the patient because the patient did nothing wrong. No matter who they had in there, it is important to practice careful hygienic practices because of diseases that can be transmitted from patient to patient. I made a special note that whenever the nursing staff came into the room, they always wore rubber gloves. They were clearly concerned for themselves and not the patients. If current investigation did not substantiate unhygienic conditions, then this is a bonus for the current patients. What I complained about *did* happen. There is no way that anyone in their right minds could have found the conditions acceptable under any circumstances. The question remains: Did the supervisors admit that there was "urine" on the toilet seat that did not belong to me and I was expected to use the toilet seat in question?

Allegation #3: I stand by my original allegation. Your findings clearly were the most disturbing.... It is troubling to react to what is written.... May I strongly recommend that your findings alone be shown to doctors who are thoroughly familiar with Sickle Cell pain and ask if they would characterize a crisis using the words: yelling, uncooperative, argumentative, noncompliant, argue, etc. These accounts are a complete fabrication and an insult to anyone in my condition. What is the correct behavior for someone in severe pain? I have never in my life uttered, "I don't care about anyone else. You need to take care of me." Those are words made up by the nurse. (That is not how I speak!) The physician's account of what she asked me, "I asked pt if she takes any narcotic pain medication at home" is a complete *lie*. What she did was add an "s" to narcotics and left off the "pain medication." Her statement should read, "Tell me Mrs. Johnson, are you taking any narcotics at home? That's a legitimate medical question," and she repeated the question. Again, I am asking your board a definitive question: Is what is described in this paragraph by your findings an acceptable characterization of a Sickle Cell Patient in crisis? And is it acceptable for a physician or any medical personnel to discuss the potential "demise" of one patient with another patient? The paragraph that states that "... she prefers to be admitted..." This statement alone should have raised eyebrows among the medical staff. As sick as I was...I would later receive four pints of blood as an inpatient. Does this mean that the doctor would have sent me home if I had "preferred" to go home rather than be admitted? How could this have been justified for someone in my condition?

And my response to the hospital's top administrator:

I am well aware that your hospital had no role in the preparation of this report. However, there are statements clearly stated that have been attributed to one of your doctors and a nurse that should have been disturbing to you as an administrator and in which the general public would be greatly concerned. Those were absolutely lies. I want to know how you have addressed those allegations with the employees in question.

I again ask the question: "Do you support this type of description for a Sickle Cell Patient in crisis?" How can the general public trust the medical profession if this is how they are being permitted to portray their patients?

I will disagree with the timeliness that you have described. However, the major issue here is not how soon I was triaged but the attitude and disrespect that accompanied the anguish that a crisis put me in.

In (all) my years of existence, I had never had a question of this nature posed in that manner. "Tell me Mrs. Johnson, are you taking any narcotics at home," accompanied with insulting body language will never be forgotten. I note that you are apologizing for the way I felt... I want you to apologize because you *understood* that it was absolutely wrong. The implications are clear: You view me as a dope addict! How is it that no other physician that I have been in contact with has ever asked me such a question in that manner? Given my medical history, I think you will agree that I perhaps have been in contact with lots of doctors along the way.... Of course medical providers need to know what medications you are/have taken so as not to risk negative reactions or overdose. Doctors have always asked "Are you taking any medication at home and/or did you take any medication before coming to the hospital?" and then they would proceed to write down the name of whatever it is the patient told them. Can you not understand how it reached my brain, as "here is another dope addict?"

I did not need to be told that another patient was dying. Does this mean that it is okay to discuss one patient's situation with another patient? Did the staff explain to other patients that I was a dope addict needing a fix or a sickle cell patient in crisis? My situation had nothing to do with the order in which patients were seen. My situation was uncontrollable. While I waited to be treated, what was I to do? Not cry? Not scream due to the severity of the pain? Specifically, how was I to behave that would have been acceptable?

I would like to redirect your attention to the comments attributed to your medical staff during the investigation. No amount of sensitivity training is going to substitute for lack of common sense... for the nurse to state that I said, "I don't care about anyone but me... You must take care of me...etc. is downright stupid. If I am in all that pain, how am I able to carry on such conversations? Please advise under what circumstances the CEO meets with those in the community that have concerns about the product his staff produces?

If doctors and other medical professionals would take the time to understand sickle cell disease and the struggles a patient faces daily, they would be unlikely to behave in such an insulting and condescending manner. To imply that I might have taken narcotics at home they would be unlikely to behave cut to the core of my very being.

The following is the final response from the CMS Health Quality Center regarding my complaint arising from the overdose:

…Unfortunately, (blank) Hospital has not provided us with a complete medical record so we are unable to proceed with our review at this time. (Blank) has taken the appropriate steps as mandated by the Centers for Medicare & Medicaid (CMS) at this time to address the issue. Your case, therefore, has been closed until a copy of the entire medical record is received.

Should the facility provide us with a copy of the entire medical record, we will reopen the case and begin our review of your stated complaint. If this occurs, I will contact you in writing, rather than by telephone, per your prior request to receive only written communications updates.

We appreciate your contacting us, and we will contact you in the future with updated information should the facility send a copy of the medical record to us.

This response implies that the hospital has the option of providing information or not providing information. In other words, they can thumb their noses at their patients. These issues beg for lawyers willing to work pro bono on behalf of patients. The average patient cannot begin to fight alone for a successful resolution.

Chapter Ten
The Power Within

"Power travels in the bloodlines, handed out before birth.

Louise Erdrich

Tears are often perceived as a weakness. For sickle cell patients, however, they are also a sign of strength. After we have a good cry, we feel a renewed burst of adrenalin that builds a protective wall to prepare us for the next pain episode. Until there is a cure, we will shed tears. A sudden outburst of tears is likely to startle those nearest us to the point where they feel helpless and unsure how to assist us.

Our strength shines through time and time again. We remain standing. We continue to fight until there is no more fight in us. The pain that we have endured has been so great that an amputation of our affected limbs would have been welcome.

In hospital emergency rooms, where we frequent often, we face long wait times, the risk of infectious disease, and a lack of compassion. While these issues are all important, we sickle cell patients are most concerned with the dearth of compassion in our interactions with medical professionals.

Sickle cell disease is hereditary. There is no cure. Our primary care doctors won't cure us. Therefore, at the very least we expect compassion from the medical professionals treating us.

The lack of compassion is a common complaint of sickle cell patients throughout the world. Sickle cell forums exist all over the world for patients and families to express their fears, concerns, and hopes for the future. These forums offer emotional support. They allow us to trade stories about our treatment and experiences with pain. If medical professionals would monitor these discussions, perhaps they would understand the deep hurt inflicted upon us by the insinuation that we are drug addicts seeking a fix.

Our screams of agony should speed up our treatment, not hinder it. We cannot control the level of pain that we experience. Many sickle cell patients have sought relief from their pain by relocating around the world seeking improved and compassionate treatment from those who seem to have a genuine interest in treating us. People flock to doctors and medical facilities who have established themselves as a part of the caring profession.

To feel compassion is to recognize another person's suffering; to want to relieve that pain and remove the cause of that distress. One caring physician once wrote that in the art of healing, compassion is the force that sets knowledge into motion. Sickle cell patients need more medical professionals with a thirst for knowledge about the disease.

Compassion has seemingly disappeared. Healing has become a business. Doctors spend more of their time speaking the languages of insurance companies and government bureaucrats than in terms of treatment and care. There are also the added demands of electronic recordkeeping, busier and more extended schedules, and growing patient loads. Some doctors fail to recognize the importance of humility in practicing medicine.

Our first contact with medical professionals is usually the emergency room. Unfortunately, too many emergency rooms are staffed with doctors at different stages in their careers. The myriad of challenges are certain to be overwhelming at times. For this very reason, the emergency rooms have two choices: (1) make a conscious effort to rotate the most experienced medical staff throughout this department seven days a week, twenty-four hours a day or (2) be extremely careful in selecting the person in charge of that department.

Because of the way I structured or failed to structure my life in the beginning, I did not begin to understand what this illness was all about until I was well into my fifties. I did not have a vision of my future. I was always in a survival mode. Reflecting on my life up to that point, I now understand quite well why there was no family or friends to accompany me to the hospital. Sickle cell anemia simply was not talked about or discussed in any meaningful way. Therefore, I never had anyone on standby.

As a patient, I did not know how to explain what was happening to me. I only knew that I was subject to sudden excruciating episodes and there seemed to be no one who could make it go away forever. When not in pain, I was usually tired. I had not made the connection between sickle cell anemia and fatigue. Therefore, I said nothing. I just retreated into my own world of silence. I was not going to try to explain my fatigue to those who viewed me as purely lazy.

Because of my vast experiences with emergency rooms in many localities, I would like to pass on words of wisdom to those who are traveling down the same road. To have someone accompany you to the hospital is not enough. They need to understand your condition and know what to do when they get there.

As sickle cell patients, we have to create our own caring, nurturing treatment environments. As stated in the previous chapter, I have had more than my share of inappropriate treatment at the hands of those who were supposed to be caring for me. What the medical professionals did not know or seem to understand was the sheer will on my part to survive.

As I've chronicled in these pages, I carried my fight against sickle cell disease into all arenas of my life. My battle reached a culmination when I finally had enough and began to challenge the hospitals and their staff on what I considered their rude, insensitive, and unprofessional treatment. That treatment prompted me to write this book. Writing this book is one of the biggest victories of my journey.

Epilogue

For the first fifteen years of my life, I was treated only with liniment. After my diagnosis with sickle cell anemia at the age of sixteen, I received an initial blood transfusion in the doctor's office in Jacksonville, Florida. Thereafter, whenever a crisis would occur, the treatment was a blood transfusion. I don't ever remember any specific medicine that was prescribed at those times. As a result of many transfusions and crises, I eventually developed hypertension, kidney disease, and liver concerns. In June 2011, I had my left shoulder replaced and in May 2013, my right shoulder was replaced. In recent years (since my sixties), I have been taking several medications.

I am now receiving a Procit™ shot biweekly. This helps my body produce red blood cells. The medicine has increased my energy level, which has also increased my quality of life.

The one recommendation that I do question was being prescribed Vitron-C™, especially with my history of blood transfusions. Multiple blood transfusions may lead to too much iron in one's blood. This can damage parts of one's body, including the liver and heart. Vitron-C™ is a high potency dietary iron supplement. Perhaps a doctor who reads this can provide me an answer.

Being a sickle cell anemia patient can be expensive. My liver damage had progressed to the point where at one time, I was taking medicine (Exjade™) – which costs in excess of $5,000 a month – to lower my level of Ferratin. Ferratin is a protein that stores and releases iron. High levels of Ferratin can signal iron overload. My monthly prescription costs are now in the hundreds of dollars.

I hope this book will serve as a start to what will come next and continue the discussion of sickle cell disease as we continue this fight for equity, acceptance and dignity.

About the Author

Judy Gray Johnson has been living with sickle cell for more than 70 years. She has nearly 40 years of experience in public education, having taught elementary, middle and high school in Virginia and Maryland. Ms. Johnson holds a Master's Degree in Special Education from Virginia State University, in Petersburg, Virginia, and a Bachelor's Degree in Elementary Education from South Carolina State University in Orangeburg, South Carolina. She is also certified in the Commonwealth of Virginia as an Elementary and Secondary School Principal. For three years, she served as president of the Fairfax County Federation of Teachers (the second-largest teachers union in the state of Virginia) representing teachers and aides in the largest school district in the state of Virginia.

Ms. Johnson is the author of two other books on sickle cell: *Living with Sickle Cell Disease: the Struggle to Survive* and *Resilience: A Personal Story of Coping with the Ravages of Sickle Cell Disease...Against All Odds*. Ms. Johnson lives in Valencia, California, and continues to advocate in the cause of finding real quality of life changes for those suffering with sickle cell.

She is in the "throws" of her next life by writing and speaking to groups. A children's book is next in her future. Ms. Johnson is available to speak to school groups and organizations by contacting her at jgjproductions@gmail.com.

Facts

What is Sickle Cell Disease?

Sickle Cell Disease (SCD) is a group of inherited red blood cell disorders.

- Healthy red blood cells are round, and they move through small blood vessels to carry oxygen to all parts of the body.
- In SCD, the red blood cells become hard and sticky and look like a C-shaped farm tool called a "sickle."
- Sickle cells die early, which causes a constant shortage of red blood cells.
- Sickle cells can get stuck and clog the blood flow of blood and oxygen to organs in the body. These blockages cause repeated episodes of severe pain, organ damage, serious infections, or even stroke.

What Causes Sickle Cell Disease?

SCD is inherited in the same way that people get the color of their eyes, skin and hair.

- A person with SCD is born with it.
- People cannot catch SCD from being around a person who has it.

Who is Affected By Sickle Cell Disease?

- It is estimated that SCD affects 90,000 to 100,000 people in the United States, mainly Blacks or African Americans.
- The disease occurs among about 1 of every 500 Black or African American births and among about 1 out of every 36,000 Hispanic-American births.

- SCD affects millions of people throughout the world and is particularly common among those whose ancestors come from sub-Saharan Africa; regions in the Western Hemisphere (South America, the Caribbean, and Central America); Saudi Arabia; India; and Mediterranean countries such as Turkey, Greece and Italy.

- **Types of SCD**

  Following are the most common types of SCD:

  ### HbSS

  People who have this form of SCD inherit two sickle cell genes ("S"), one from each parent. This is commonly called SICKLE CELL ANEMIA and is usually the most severe form of the disease.

  ### HbSC

  People who have this form of SCD inherit a sickle cell gene ("S") from one parent and from the other parent a gene for an abnormal hemoglobin called "C". Hemoglobin is a protein that allows red blood cells to carry oxygen to all parts of the body. This is usually a milder form of SCD.

  ### HbS beta Thalassemia

  People who have this form of SCD inherit one sickle cell gene ("S") from one parent and one gene for beta thalassemia, another type of anemia, from the other parent.

  There are two types of beta thalassemia: "0" and "+." Those with HbS beta 0-thalassemia usually have a severe form of SCD. People with HbS beta +-thalassemia tend to have a milder form of SCD.
  There are also a few rare types of SCD:
  HbSD, HbSE, and HbSO

  People who have these forms of SCD, inherit one sickle cell gene ("S") and one gene from an abnormal type of hemoglobin ("D", "E", or "O"). Hemoglobin is a protein that allows red blood cells to carry oxygen to all parts of the body. The severity of these rarer types of SCD varies.

Sickle Cell Trait (SCT)

HbAS
People who have SCT, inherit one sickle cell gene ("S") from one parent and one normal gene ("A") from the other parent. This is called SICKLE CELL TRAIT (SCT). People with SCT usually do not have any of the signs of the disease and live a normal life, but they can pass the trait on to their children. Additionally, there are a few, uncommon health problems that may potentially be related to SCT.

Cause of SCD
SCD is a genetic condition that is present at birth. It is inherited when a child receives two sickle cell genes, one from each parent.

Diagnosis

SCD is diagnosed with a simple blood test. It most often is found at birth during routine newborn screening tests at the hospital. In addition, SCD can be diagnosed before birth.

Because children with SCD are at an increased risk of infection and other health problems, early diagnosis and treatment are important.

You can call your local sickle cell organization to find out how to get tested.

Anemia (low blood): A condition in which there is less haemoglobin in the blood than usual so that the blood can't carry as much oxygen.

Dehydration: A condition caused by not having enough water in the body. Dehydration can happen with diarrhea, fever or exercise. It may cause a sickling episode in someone with SCD.

Inherited: A characteristic passed on from parents to their children. Sickle cell disease is an inherited disease.

Leg Ulcer: A breakage in the skin that begins as a small sore on the lower leg – above, over and around the ankle. It can be caused by injury and decreased blood flow.

Priapism: A persistent, painful, unwanted erection of the penis caused by sickling.

Spleen: An organ on the left side of the body that may be felt below the rib cage. It is a filter to remove bacteria from the blood. This organ does not work well in sickle cell disease. It can trap blood and become enlarged.

What Health Problems Does Sickle Cell Disease Cause?

Following are some of the most common complications of SCD:

"Pain Episode" or "Crisis": Sickle cells don't move easily through small blood vessels and can get stuck and clog blood flow. This causes pain that can start suddenly, be mild to server, and last for any length of time.

Infection: People with SCD, especially infants and children, are more likely to experience harmful infections such as flu, meningitis and hepatitis.

Hand-Foot Syndrome: Swelling in the hands and feet, often along with a fever, is caused by the sickle cells getting stuck in the blood vessels and blocking the blood from flowing freely through the hands and feet.

Eye Disease: SCD can affect the blood vessels in the eye and lead to long term damage.

Acute Chest Syndrome (ACS): Blockage of the flow of blood to the lungs can cause acute chest syndrome. ACS is similar to pneumonia; symptoms include chest pain, coughing, difficulty breathing and fever. It can be life threatening and should be treated in a hospital.

Stroke: Sickle cells can clog blood flow to the brain and cause a stroke. A stroke can result in lifelong disabilities and learning problems.

Complications and Treatments

People with SCD start to have signs of the disease during the first year of life, usually around 5 months of age. Symptoms and complications of SCD are different for each person and can range from mild to severe.

There is no single best treatment for all people with SCD. Treatment options are different for each person depending on the symptoms.

Cure

The only cure for SCD is bone marrow or stem cell transplant.

Bone marrow is a soft, fatty tissue inside the center of the bones where blood cells are made. A bone marrow or stem cell transplant is a procedure that takes healthy cells that form blood from one person, the donor, and puts them into someone whose bone marrow is not working properly.

Bone marrow or stem cell transplants are very risky, and can have serious side effects, including death. For the transplant to work, the bone marrow must be a close match. Usually, the best donor is a brother or sister. Bone marrow or stem cell transplants are used only in cases of severe SCD for children who have minimal organ damage from the disease.

Acute Chest Syndrome (ACS): Blockage of the flow of blood to the lungs can cause acute chest syndrome. ACS is similar to pneumonia; symptoms include chest pain, coughing, difficulty breathing and fever. It can be life threatening and should be treated in a hospital.

Stroke: Sickle cells can clog blood flow to the brain and cause a stroke. A stroke can result in lifelong disabilities and learning problems.

Source: CDC- Centers for Disease Control & Prevention

http://www.cdc.gov/ncbddd/sicklecell/facts.html

Resources

National Resource Directory
http://www.cdc.gov/ncbddd/sicklecell/map/map-nationalresourcedirectory.html

The Sickle Cell Disease National Resource Directory is a listing of national agencies, specialty care centers, and community-based organizations that provide services and resources for people affected by sickle cell disease (SCD). The goal of this directory is to help people find SCD services and resources. The information from this directory is sorted by state. Within each state, the resources are listed by type: Providers/Sickle Cell Centers, Non-Profits/Associations/Foundations, and Support Groups. In many cases, organizations offer both clinical and non-clinical resources and services. When making contact, ask about other services that may be offered such as support groups and social services.

Everyone must be accountable to someone else. In the event of an issue with medical care, it is much more effective to go up the chain of command. Give people opportunities to correct any problems. For example, issues arising from treatment in emergency rooms should be reported to the emergency room physician of record.

If the situation has not been resolved to your satisfaction, then report it to the supervisor of the emergency room physician. If the situation is still unresolved, report it to the head administrator of the hospital. In the event it is still unresolved, then send a complaint to the board of directors of that hospital. This gives everyone an opportunity to get themselves on record for appropriately handling a situation. Should the issue still not be resolved to your satisfaction, then go outside the hospital and contact the state medical board that regulates the performances of doctors and nurses within that state.

There are many resources available for further information on sickle cell disease. Please note that the information provided by these organizations, government agencies, and websites is for educational purposes only. For specific medical advice, diagnoses, and treatment, consult your physician. The physical and website addresses listed are current as of this writing and are subject to change.

National Health Service Sickle Cell and Thalasseaemia Screeing Programme
http://www.sct.screening.nhs.uk - For A downloadable copy of *A Parent's Guide to Care and Management of Your Child with Sickle Cell Disease*

SCOOTER Open Education Resources for Sickle Cell and Thalassaemia
http://www.sicklecellanaemia.org - For free sickle cell/thalassaemia images and other open educational resources

Organizations:

Sickle Cell Disease Association of America
231 E. Baltimore Street Suite 800
Baltimore, MD 21202
(410) 528-1555
http://www.sicklecelldisease.org.

Advocacy group whose mission is to advocate for and enhance its membership's ability to improve the quality of health, life and services for individuals, families, and communities affected by sickle cell disease and related conditions, while promoting the search for a cure for all people in the world with sickle cell disease.

The Joint Commission
One Renaissance Boulevard

Oakbrook Terrace, IL 60181
(800) 994-6610
complaint@jointcommission.org www.jointcommission.org

Accepts complaints of poor hospital treatment and uses the information to identify non-compliance with accreditation or certification standards for hospitals.

Government Agencies:

National Heart, Lung and Blood Institute
P.O. Box 30105
Bethesda, MD 20824
(301) 592-8573
http://www.nhlbi.nih.gov/health/health-topics/topics/sca

National Institute of Health sub-agency that provides information on sickle cell disease and global leadership for a research, training, and education program to promote the prevention and treatment of heart, lung, and blood diseases and to enhance the health of all individuals so that they can live longer and more fulfilling lives.

Centers for Disease Control
600 Clifton Road
Atlanta, GA 30333
(800) 232-4636
http://www.cdc.gov/ncbddd/sicklecell/index.html

Department of Health and Human Services sub-agency collaborates to create the expertise, information and tools that people and communities need to protect their health – through health promotion, prevention of disease, injury and disability, and preparedness for new health threats.

United States Department of Justice
Civil Rights Division

Disability Rights Section - NYA
950 Pennsylvania Avenue NW
Washington, DC 20530
(800) 514-0301
www.ada.gov

Provides information about the Americans with Disabilities Act, which prohibits employers from discriminating against people with disabilities in application procedures, hiring, firing, promotions, pay and training. (To contact an attorney, search the Internet via such search engines as Google, Bing, or Yahoo for "Americans with Disabilities Act Lawyers and Law Firms by State of Province.")

The Disability Rights Section provides information about the Americans with Disabilities Act, which prohibits employers from discriminating against people with disabilities in application procedures, hiring, firing, promotions, pay and training. (To contact an attorney, search the Internet via such search engines as Google, Bing, Yahoo for "Americans with Disabilities Act Lawyers and Law Firms by State or Province.")

Websites:

Department of Pain Medicine & Palliative Care at Beth Israel Medical Center in New York
http://www.stoppain.org/pain_medicine/content/chronicpain/sickle.asp

Medicine.Net, an online, healthcare media publishing company:
http://www.medicinetnet.com/sickle_cell/article.htm

The Sickle Cell Information Center
http://www.scinfo.org

Sickle Cell Disease: Kids Health by Nemours: (Page)

http://www.kidshealth.org/teen/diseases_conditions/blood/sickle_cell_a nemia.html

Sickle Cell Warriors

http://www.sicklecellwarriors.com